# Medical Issues in Boxing

*Guest Editors*

GERARD P. VARLOTTA, DO, FACSM
BARRY D. JORDAN, MD, MPH, FACSM

# CLINICS IN
# SPORTS MEDICINE

www.sportsmed.theclinics.com

*Consulting Editor*
MARK D. MILLER, MD

October 2009 • Volume 28 • Number 4

SAUNDERS an imprint of ELSEVIER, Inc.

**W.B. SAUNDERS COMPANY**
*A Division of Elsevier Inc.*

1600 John F. Kennedy Blvd. • Suite 1800 • Philadelphia, Pennsylvania 19103

http://www.theclinics.com

**CLINICS IN SPORTS MEDICINE Volume 28, Number 4**
**October 2009 ISSN 0278-5919, ISBN-13: 978-1-4377-1276-6, ISBN-10: 1-4377-1276-2**

Editor: Ruth Malwitz
Developmental Editor: Donald Mumford

*Clinics in Sports Medicine* (ISSN 0278-5919) is published quarterly by Elsevier Inc., 360 Park Avenue South, New York, NY 10010-1710. Months of publication are January, April, July, and October. Application to mail at periodicals postage rates is pending at New York, NY and at additional mailing offices. Subscription prices are $253.00 per year (US individuals), $393.00 per year (US institutions), $127.00 per year (US students), $286.00 per year (Canadian individuals), $475.00 per year (Canadian institutions), $177.00 (Canadian students), $347.00 per year (foreign individuals), $475.00 per year (foreign institutions), and $177.00 per year (foreign students). Foreign air speed delivery is included in all *Clinics* subscription prices. All prices are subject to change without notice. **POSTMASTER:** Send address changes to *Clinics in Sports Medicine*, Elsevier Health Sciences Division, Subscription Customer Service, 3251 Riverport Lane, Maryland Heights, MO 63043. Customer Service (orders, claims, online, change of address): Elsevier Health Sciences Division, Subscription Customer Service, 3251 Riverport Lane, Maryland Heights, MO 63043. Tel: 1-800-654-2452 (U.S. and Canada); 314-447-8871(outside U.S. and Canada). Fax: 314-447-8029. E-mail: journalscustomerservice-usa@elsevier.com (for print support); journalsonlinesupport-usa@elsevier.com (for online support).

*Reprints.* For copies of 100 or more of articles in this publication, please contact the Commercial Reprints Department, Elsevier Inc., 360 Park Avenue South, New York, NY 10010-1710. Tel.: 212-633-3812; Fax: 212-462-1935; E-mail: reprints@elsevier.com.

*Clinics in Sports Medicine* is covered in *MEDLINE/PubMed (Index Medicus) Current Contents/Clinical Medicine, Excerpta Medica,* and *ISI/Biomed.*

# Contributors

## CONSULTING EDITOR

**MARK D. MILLER, MD**
S. Ward Casscells Professor of Orthopaedic Surgery, University of Virginia; Team Physician, James Madison University, Charlottesville, Virginia

## GUEST EDITORS

**GERARD P. VARLOTTA, DO, FACSM**
Clinical Associate Professor, Department of Rehabilitation Medicine, New York University School of Medicine, Rusk Institute of Rehabilitation Medicine, New York, New York

**BARRY D. JORDAN, MD, MPH, FACSM**
Director, Brain Injury Program, Burke Rehabilitation Hospital, White Plains, New York; Associate Professor of Clinical Neurology, Department of Neurology, Weill Medical College of Cornell University, New York, New York; Former Medical Director/Chief Medical Officer, New York State Athletic Commission, New York, New York

## AUTHORS

**STEVEN BELDNER, MD**
Assistant Professor, Department of Orthopaedic Surgery, Albert Einstein College of Medicine, Hand Surgery Center, Beth Israel Medical Center, New York, New York

**DOMENIC F. COLETTA, Jr., MD**
Chief Ringside Physician, New Jersey State Athletic Control Board, Trenton, New Jersey; Executive Sr. Vice-President, American Association of Professional Ringside Physicians, Darien, Connecticut; Cape Emergency Physicians, Department of Medicine, Cape Regional Medical Center, Cape May Court House, New Jersey

**GUSTAVO CORRALES, MD**
Cornea Fellow, Department of Cornea and Refractive Surgery, New York Eye and Ear Infirmary, New York, New York

**ANTHONY CURRERI, MD**
Assistant Professor, Ophthalmology Department, New York Eye and Ear Infirmary, New York, New York

**STEVEN FLANAGAN, MD**
Professor and Chairman, Department of Rehabilitation Medicine, New York University School of Medicine, Rusk Institute of Rehabilitation Medicine, New York, New York

**BARRY D. JORDAN, MD, MPH, FACSM**
Director, Brain Injury Program, Burke Rehabilitation Hospital, White Plains, New York; Associate Professor of Clinical Neurology, Department of Neurology, Weill Medical College of Cornell University; Former Medical Director/Chief Medical Officer, New York State Athletic Commission, New York, New York

**MICHAEL KELLY, DO**
Ringside Physician, Procare Medical Associates, Livingston, New Jersey

**OSRIC S. KING, MD**
Chief Medical Officer, New York State Athletic Commission; Assistant Attending Sports Medicine, Hospital for Special Surgery, New York, New York

**TODD LEFKOWITZ, DO**
Clinical Instructor, Department of Rehabilitation Medicine, New York University School of Medicine, Rusk Institute of Rehabilitation Medicine, New York, New York

**CHARLES P. MELONE, Jr., MD**
Clinical Professor, Department of Orthopaedic Surgery, Albert Einstein College of Medicine; and Chief, Hand Surgery Center, Beth Israel Medical Center, New York, New York

**DANIEL B. POLATSCH, MD**
Assistant Professor, Department of Orthopaedic Surgery, Albert Einstein College of Medicine, Hand Surgery Center, Beth Israel Medical Center, New York, New York

**MICHAEL B. SCHWARTZ, DO**
Chairman, American Association of Professional Ringside Physicians (AAPRP), Darien Connecticut; Chief Ringside Physician, Mohegan Sun Department of Athletic Regulations, Uncasville, Connecticut; Chief Ringside Physician, Mashantucket Pequot Tribal Nation Athletic Commission, Mashantucket, Connecticut; Internist – Board Certified ABIM, Associated Internists of Darien, Darien, Connecticut; Associate Professor of Medicine, Norwalk Hospital, Norwalk, Connecticut; Clinical Instructor, Department of Medicine, Yale University Hospital, New Haven, Connecticut; Adjunct Assistant Professor of Medicine, New York Medical College, Valhalla, New York

**STEPHEN A. SIEGEL, MD, FACC, FACSM**
Clinical Assistant Professor, Department of Medicine, Leon H. Charney Division of Cardiology, New York University School of Medicine; President, Greater New York Regional Chapter, American College of Sports Medicine, New York, New York.

**GERARD VARLOTTA, DO, FACSM**
Clinical Associate Professor, Department of Rehabilitation Medicine, New York University School of Medicine, Rusk Institute of Rehabilitation Medicine, New York, New York

**GARY I. WADLER, MD, FACP, FACSM**
Clinical Associate Professor of Medicine, NYU School of Medicine, Manhasset, New York; Chairman, Prohibited List and Methods Committee, World Anti-doping Agency (WADA), Montreal, Quebec, Canada

# Contents

**Foreword**                                                                                           ix

Mark D. Miller

**Preface**                                                                                            xi

Gerard P. Varlotta and Barry Jordan

**Medical Safety in Boxing: Administrative, Ethical, Legislative, and Legal
Considerations**                                                                                      505

Michael B. Schwartz

> The roles and responsibilities of the ringside physician are complex and
> have evolved into a unique specialty in sport medicine. In addition to the
> medical aspects of ringside medicine, the doctor is now responsible for
> many administrative, ethical, and legal considerations. This article reviews
> and details the numerous roles the ringside physician plays in the sport of
> boxing.

**Role of the Ringside Physician and Medical Preparticipation Evaluation
of Boxers**                                                                                           515

Michael Kelly

> Ringside physicians play a dynamic and multifaceted role in combat
> sports. Extensive preparation and long hours are required. This article re-
> views prelicensing, prebout, and postbout evaluations. It also outlines
> some crucial decision-making and actions necessary during the event, in-
> cluding rendering of instant medical opinions on bout termination and
> acute care of the injured fighter.

**Cardiovascular Issues in Boxing and Contact Sports**                                                521

Stephen A. Siegel

> Despite the inherent risks associated with exercise in general and boxing
> in particular, the sport has had a limited number of catastrophic cardiovas-
> cular events. Screening should be based on risks involved and become
> more extensive with the advancement of the athlete. Anatomic and elec-
> trophysiologic risks need to be assessed and may preclude participation
> with resultant life style and economic complications. There should be
> adequate preparation for the rare potential cardiovascular complication
> at all events, with the ability to rapidly assess and treat arrhythmias.

**The Status of Doping and Drug Use and the Implications for Boxing**                                 533

Gary I. Wadler

> Boxers are not immune from the abuse of drugs. This article outlines the
> history of drug taking in boxing and sport in general. The current criteria

that constitute doping, and prohibited substances and methods in and out of competition, according to guidelines issued by the World Anti-Doping Agency, are listed. Drugs and therapeutic exemptions are discussed.

**Infectious Disease and Boxing**                                                          545

Osric S. King

There are no unique boxing diseases but certain factors contributing to the spread of illnesses apply strongly to the boxer, coach, and the training facility. This article examines the nature of the sport of boxing and its surrounding environment, and the likelihood of spread of infection through airborne, contact, or blood-borne routes of transmission. Evidence from other sports such as running, wrestling, and martial arts is included to help elucidate the pathophysiologic elements that could be identified in boxers.

**Brain Injury in Boxing**                                                                 561

Barry D. Jordan

Clinical decision making for injured boxers follows the same therapeutic principles as the treatment plan for other injured athletes. Just as surgical techniques have improved, so has the scientific basis for implementing therapeutic exercises progressed to return the athletes to their former level of competition.

**Nonneurologic Emergencies in Boxing**                                                    579

Domenic F. Coletta, Jr.

Professional boxing has done an admirable job in promoting safety standards in its particular sport. However, injuries occur during the normal course of competition and, unfortunately, an occasional life-threatening emergency may arise. Although most common medical emergencies in boxing are injuries from closed head trauma, in this article those infrequent but potentially catastrophic nonneurologic conditions are reviewed along with some less serious emergencies that the physician must be prepared to address.

**Eye Trauma in Boxing**                                                                   591

Gustavo Corrales and Anthony Curreri

In boxing, along with a few other sports, trauma is inherent to the nature of the sport; therefore it is considered a high-risk sport for ocular injuries. The long-term morbidity of ocular injuries suffered by boxers is difficult to estimate due to the lack of structured long-term follow-up of these athletes. Complications of blunt ocular trauma may develop years after the athlete has retired from the ring and is no longer considered to be at risk for boxing-related injuries. This article describes the wide range of eye injuries a boxer can sustain, and their immediate and long-term clinical management.

**Disabling Hand Injuries in Boxing: Boxer's Knuckle and Traumatic Carpal Boss**    **609**

Charles P. Melone, Jr., Daniel B. Polatsch, and Steven Beldner

> This article describes the treatment of the two most debilitating hand-related boxing injuries: boxer's knuckle and traumatic carpal boss. Recognition of the normal anatomy as well as the predictable pathology facilitates an accurate diagnosis and precision surgery. For boxer's knuckle, direct repair of the disrupted extensor hood, without the need for tendon augmentation, has been consistently employed; for traumatic carpal boss, arthrodesis of the destabilized carpometacarpal joints has been the preferred method of treatment. Precisely executed operative treatment of both injuries has resulted in a favorable outcome, as in the vast majority of cases the boxers have experienced relief of pain, restoration of function, and an unrestricted return to competition.

**Rehabilitation of Orthopaedic and Neurologic Boxing Injuries**    **623**

Todd Lefkowitz, Steven Flanagan, and Gerard Varlotta

> Clinical decision making for injured boxers follows the same therapeutic principles as the treatment plan for other injured athletes. Just as surgical techniques have improved, so has the scientific basis for implementing therapeutic exercises progressed to return the athletes to their former level of competition.

**Index**    **641**

FORTHCOMING ISSUES

*January 2010*
**Rehabilitation from the Athletic Trainer's/Physical Trainer's Perspective**
Jeff G. Konin, PhD, ATC, PT,
*Guest Editor*

*April 2010*
**Rehabilitation from the Orthopedic Surgeon's Perspective**
Claude T. Moorman, III, MD,
*Guest Editor*

*July 2010*
**The Runner**
Robert Wilder, MD, *Guest Editor*

*October 2010*
**The Athlete's Elbow**
Marc R. Safran, MD, *Guest Editor*

RECENT ISSUES

*October 2009*
**Obesity and Diabetes in Sports Medicine**
Susan E. Kirk, MD and
Dilaawar J. Mistry, MD, MS, ATC,
*Guest Editors*

*April 2009*
**Allografts**
Darren L. Johnson, MD, *Guest Editor*

*January 2009*
**Future Trends in Sports Medicine**
Scott A. Rodeo, MD, *Guest Editor*

*October 2008*
**Shoulder Problems in Athletes**
Benjamin Shaffer, MD, *Guest Editor*

**THE CLINICS ARE NOW AVAILABLE ONLINE!**

Access your subscription at:
**www.theclinics.com**

# Foreword

Although we have until now largely refrained from producing sports-specific topics, we elected here to devote an issue to boxing because of the unique nature of this sport and the sometimes devastating injuries associated with it. Drs. Varlotta and Jordan have done a great job of putting this issue together.

As you would expect, head injuries are very common in boxing, and much of the issue is devoted to this topic. The editors did not stop there, however, and also included several insightful articles on the role of the physician, safety, doping concerns, and a plethora of medical topics. The result is an excellent treatise for the physician who covers this challenging sport, and for all of us who share a common interest in taking care of athletes.

Mark D. Miller, MD
James Madison University
400 Ray C. Hunt Dr, Suite 330, Charlottesville, VA 22908-0159

E-mail address:
mdm3p@virginia.edu (M.D. Miller)

Clin Sports Med 28 (2009) ix
doi:10.1016/j.csm.2009.08.001          **sportsmed.theclinics.com**

# Preface

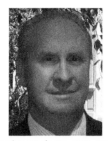 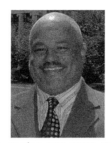

Gerard P. Varlotta, DO, FACSM    Barry Jordan, MD, MPH, FACSM
*Guest Editors*

Medical injuries are the unfortunate consequence of all sports but the prevalence is higher in combative sports participation. In boxing, injuries can be found crossing the standard lines of medical care and include neurologic, ophthalmologic, musculoskeletal, and behavioral. The ringside physician needs to be aware and capable of handling all emergent neurologic and non-neurologic aspects of the sport for the protection of the participants. Unanticipated catastrophic occurrences need to be minimized through education of the medical aspects of the sport and knowledge of the sport itself.

This issue of the *Clinics of Sports Medicine* is a comprehensive accumulation of the variety of issues that need to be recognized by those participating in the health care of boxers to ensure their safety. It is not intended to be a complete in-depth analysis on each aspect but is meant to provide a basis for further learning to ensure the safety of the participants. This issue will discuss the administrative and legal issues, and the pre-participation assessment, as well as the acute and nonacute neurologic, ophthalmologic, facial, infectious disease, cardiac, orthopedic, and rehabilitation treatment of the injured boxer. Additionally, an understanding of the state of performance enhancement in sports and its relevance to boxing is also included.

"Medical Issues in Boxing" concentrates on the sport-specific issues that concern those participating in the medical care of the boxer. Rehabilitation and injury prophylaxis is the next level of achievement that will provide a better understanding of the risks associated with the sport. A better national tracking system of injuries and the long-term sequelae is necessary to continue to improve the safety of participation in the sport of boxing.

Gerard P. Varlotta, DO, FACSM
Department of Rehabilitation Medicine
New York University School of Medicine
Rusk Institute of Rehabilitation Medicine
317 East 34th Street, 5th Floor
New York, NY 10016, USA

Clin Sports Med 28 (2009) xi–xii
doi:10.1016/j.csm.2009.08.002
0278-5919/09/$ – see front matter © 2009 Elsevier Inc. All rights reserved.

Barry Jordan, MD, MPH, FACSM
Brain Injury Program
Burke Rehabilitation Hospital
785 Mamaroneck Avenue
White Plains, NY 10603, USA

E-mail addresses:
gerard.varlotta@nyumc.org (G.P. Varlotta)
bjordan@burke.org (B. Jordan)

# Medical Safety in Boxing: Administrative, Ethical, Legislative, and Legal Considerations

Michael B. Schwartz, DO[a,b,c,d,e,f,g,*]

**KEYWORDS**

- Boxing Safety • Administrative • Medical • Ethical
- Legislative • Legal Considerations

## ADMINISTRATIVE

The ringside physician is not only responsible for safety of the fighter during a contest but is responsible for the pre- and post-fight evaluations as well.

### Pre-Participation Examination

The pre-participation examination is the most vital aspect in determining the fitness of the fighter, thus reducing the risk of death and minimizing injuries. This examination includes completion of a comprehensive medical history form. The form should be simple and concise, and identify pertinent issues. For convenience, it should be available in both English and Spanish; however, regardless of spoken language an interpreter should be available to assist the fighter in completing the form. The form should then be reviewed by the examining physician and signed by both the fighter and doctor.

The actual pre-fight physical examination affords the ringside physician an opportunity to identify issues that may put a fighter at risk for serious injury. Therefore, this

[a] American Association of Professional Ringside Physicians (AAPRP), 40 Heights Road, Suite 200, Darien, CT 06820, USA
[b] Mohegan Sun Department of Athletic Regulations, One Mohegan Sun Boulevard, Uncasville, CT 06382, USA
[c] Mashantucket Pequot Tribal Nation Athletic Commission, PO Box 3378, Mashantucket, CT 06339, USA
[d] Associated Internists of Darien, 40 Heights Road, Darien, CT 06820, USA
[e] Norwalk Hospital, 24 Stevens Street, Norwalk, CT 06850, USA
[f] Department of Medicine, Yale University Hospital, New Haven, CT, USA
[g] New York Medical College, Valhalla, NY, USA
* Norwalk Hospital, 24 Stevens Street, Norwalk, CT 06850.
*E-mail address:* ringsidemd@aol.com

Clin Sports Med 28 (2009) 505–514
doi:10.1016/j.csm.2009.06.003
0278-5919/09/$ – see front matter © 2009 Elsevier Inc. All rights reserved.

examination must take place in a quiet area and no more than 24 hours before the contest. Given the time constraints, these examinations must be performed in an efficient yet thorough manner. Thus, it is generally advisable to have a minimum of two doctors available to perform the examinations. In addition, it is recommended that the physician create a physical examination form that will serve as the official document containing the doctor's findings and evaluations.

### Minimum Medical Requirements

In 2005, the American Association of Professional Ringside Physicians (AAPRP) in cooperation with the Association of Boxing Commissions (ABC) developed the minimum suggested medical requirements for participation in boxing.[1] Although each state and tribal boxing commission may have their own set of regulations, these minimum requirements were created to standardize those tests that may identify individuals at greatest risk for injury. These tests include:

| Medical Requirements | Validity |
|---|---|
| Computed tomography (CT) scan/Magnetic resonance imaging (MRI) brain scan | Baseline |
| Dilated eye examination (ophthalmologist) | 1 y |
| Hepatitis Bs Ag, Hepatitis C Ab, Human immunodeficiency virus blood testing | 180 d |
| CT/MRI/Complete neurologic examination | 1 y |
| Electrocardiogram (with interpretation) | Initial only (if normal) |
| Complete history & physical examination | 1 y (Commission approved form) |
| Final pre-fight mini-physical | At the venue |
| Serum or urine pregnancy test | 14 d |
| Complete gynecologic examination | 6 mo |

### RINGSIDE PREPARATION

Immediately before the contest, the ringside physician and commission must confirm that final preparations are in place in the event of an emergency. These preparations must take place before every event, especially because venues frequently change. These pre-fight preparations include:

1. Meet with the team to formulate emergency plan
   Federal law mandates that an ambulance with emergency medical professionals remain on site for the duration of the event. Every ringside physician should meet with the paramedic or emergency medical technicians and formulate a plan in the event of an emergency.
2. Notify local hospital
   It is important to determine where the fighters will be sent in the event of an emergency. Ideally, it would be best to have a Level 1 trauma center available for each contest. However, boxing matches are held all over the country in cities, suburban, and rural areas. Thus, it is not always possible to have the highest level care facility nearby. Accordingly, the ringside physician and emergency medical staff should not only notify the local hospital but also identify all transport options in the event a serious injury occurs.
3. Notify on-call neurosurgeon
   After the nearest hospital for transfer of an injured fighter has been notified, it is also advisable to notify the on-call neurosurgeon that a boxing match is taking place.

This prior notification will afford the neurosurgeon an opportunity to make the necessary preparations should a boxer with a head injury be transferred to the facility.

4. Boxers' insurance forms

It is also a federal mandate that each participant be provided with health insurance for the contest. This insurance policy is secured by the promoter of the event, and a copy of the policy and information should be made available to the ringside physician before the contest. It is essential that the policy information and documentation be shared with the emergency medical personnel, the medical transport facility, and the fighter's team before the contest.

5. Ringside seating

It is advisable that each contest have a minimum of two ringside physicians attending the fight. A physician should be seated directly adjacent to the ring in each of the participants' corners. This standpoint enables the physician to observe the fighter and his or her interactions with their cornermen between rounds, and affords the doctor the opportunity to step up into the corner to evaluate a fighter should an injury arise. Ideally, a third ringside physician should be available to perform the post-fight examinations while the remaining fights on the card continue with the other two physicians at ringside.

## POST-FIGHT EXAMINATION

Each fighter should undergo a comprehensive post-fight physical examination to assess and determine the extent of injuries incurred during the bout. This examination should include an assessment of mental status and a review of all physical injuries. The findings of the examination should be reviewed with the fighter and his seconds (trainer, manager, and so forth) to assure that the evaluation and recommendations are clearly understood. A post-fight examination form should be completed and a copy of the form should be provided to both the fighter and the Commission.

The ringside physician should meet with the Commission to review injury information, suspensions, and recommendations pertaining to each fighter immediately after the bout. Finally, the ringside physician should not leave the arena until all the fighters have been evaluated and discharged from the venue.

## ETHICS

Here the ethical guidelines developed and mandated by the AAPRP for practice as a ringside physician are listed.[2]

### Ethical Guidelines for Ringside Physicians

The purpose of the Ringside Physician is to promote safety in boxing and help limit injuries to the boxer. These guidelines are set forth to help avoid conflicts of interest between the physician and other participants in boxing.

1. Any physician working at ringside must be currently licensed to practice medicine in the state in which the boxing event is taking place.
2. Physicians working at ringside may not use any illicit substances or take any drugs that may impair his or her ability to work. No use of alcohol is permitted while working at ringside.
3. Boxers may be treated in the physician's private office for conditions relating to injuries that occurred specifically from recent boxing. We discourage ringside

physicians from acting as the primary care physicians for any of the boxers, trainers, cornermen, or promoters. Doctors may perform the pre-participation physical examination or evaluate boxing-related injuries in his or her office. We encourage boxers to use ringside physicians for these examinations, as these doctors better understand the specific medical needs of these athletes.

4. Payment to physicians should be from the boxing commission and not directly from the promoter of the boxing match. The amount paid to a physician should be set in advance before the fight and we recommend that the state commissions having fees set annually based on the venue/size of the event. The fee schedule should be distributed by the state commission to the chief medical officer for the state commission and should be reviewed annually.

5. Physicians may request tickets for the boxing match directly from the boxing commission. Granting these tickets is at the sole discretion of the boxing commission. Tickets should not be requested or granted directly from a promoter.

6. No gifts may be accepted by a physician from a promoter or boxer. Autographs and photographs are permissible at the fighter's and commission's discretion.

7. As part of compensation, doctors are permitted to be reimbursed for travel and accommodations at Internal Revenue Service approved rates.

8. Ringside physicians are not permitted to place wagers on any of the fights they are working. The doctor is not allowed to divulge any information to anyone outside the normal patient-doctor confidentiality bounds set by the American Medical Association.

9. Doctors are permitted to discuss (with the media) medical issues at the end of the fight. Before or during the actual boxing match, physicians should not discuss medical conditions with nonmedical personnel or nonessential boxing personnel. Physicians are discouraged from discussing nonmedical issues, such as judges' scoring or outcomes, with the media.

10. Physicians must reveal any financial/contractual relationships with any of the boxers, promoters, or any other entity that is participating in the boxing match to the state boxing commission.

11. Ringside Physicians may act as advisors/consultants to boxing commissions, sanctioning bodies, and international bodies. They should be appropriately compensated for their work including travel and accommodation.

12. At least one physician should be at ringside during any boxing match. It is the state commission's responsibility to make certain the ringside doctor has a seat in the corner with easy access to the stairs. Physicians should be present and not leave the arena until all fighters have left the ring and have been adequately evaluated.

13. Ringside physicians are encouraged to attend boxing matches in other jurisdictions. It is our belief that increased exposure to different boxing matches and other doctors is an invaluable learning tool. Boxing commissions should provide free or discounted tickets to members of the AAPRP.

14. During AAPRP conventions or sponsored events, the AAPRP may purchase tickets from promoters at discounted rates. Promoters and other companies may sponsor AAPRP educational events with gifts or financial donations that are specifically for the event—donations should not be directly made to an individual physician.

It is recommended that all ringside physicians review these guidelines and are then asked to sign a document so that they recognize the importance of ethical behavior in the sport of boxing and agree to abide to these requirements to the best of their abilities, for example:

> *I will use my role as a ringside physician to help and care for the boxer to the best of my ability and judgment; I will abstain from harming or wrongdoing any man or woman by it. I will not violate my role as a caregiver in any fashion, will not show favoritism to any individual or organization and will maintain these ethical guidelines to support the boxer and the goal of preserving health and safety in boxing.*
> *Signature:* _____

## LEGISLATIVE

Boxing is the only major professional sport that does not have a national commission. Unlike football, which has the National Football League and baseball, which has Major League Baseball, boxing lacks a governing body to enforce its rules. As such, the congress and senate have proposed and passed federal legislation creating minimal medical requirements in professional boxing.

### The Professional Boxing Safety Act of 1996

In 1996, Congress passed the Professional Boxing Safety Act of 1996 (the Federal Boxing Act).[3,4] The stated purposes of the Federal Boxing Act are to (1) improve and expand the safety precautions that protect the welfare of professional boxers; and (2) to assist state boxing commissions to provide proper oversight for the professional boxing industry in the United States.[5] Essentially, the Federal Boxing Act has provided ringside physicians and commissions some ease in regulating the health and safety of boxers. Among other things it provides that boxers must possess federal identification cards. It also created a boxing registry to ensure that there is proper monitoring and supervision of a fighter throughout his career. Certain relevant definitions and procedures of the bill that are related to safety issues are set forth here.

#### Boxer registry
The term "boxer registry" means any entity certified by the ABC for the purposes of maintaining records and identification of boxers.

#### Physician
The term "physician" means a doctor of medicine legally authorized to practice medicine by the state in which the physician performs such function or action.

#### Suspension
The term "suspension" includes within its meaning the revocation of a boxing license.

#### Safety standards
No person may arrange, promote, organize, produce, or fight in a professional boxing match without meeting each of the following requirements or an alternative requirement in effect under regulations of a boxing commission that provides equivalent protection of the health and safety of boxers:

1. A physical examination of each boxer by a physician certifying whether or not the boxer is physically fit to safely compete, copies of which must be provided to the boxing commission.
2. Except as otherwise expressly provided under regulation of a boxing commission promulgated subsequent to October 9, 1996, an ambulance or medical personnel with appropriate resuscitation equipment continuously present on site.

3. A physician continuously present at ringside.
4. Health insurance for each boxer to provide medical coverage for any injuries sustained in the match.

### Identification card

1. Issuance: A boxing commission shall issue to each professional boxer who registers in accordance with subsection (a) of this section, an identification card that contains each of the following:
   (A) A recent photograph of the boxer.
   (B) The social security number of the boxer (or, in the case of a foreign boxer, any similar citizen identification number or professional boxer number from the country of residence of the boxer).
   (C) A personal identification number assigned to the boxer by a boxing registry.

### Procedures

Each boxing commission shall establish each of the following procedures:

1. Procedures to evaluate the professional records and physician's certification of each boxer participating in a professional boxing match in the state, and to deny authorization for a boxer to fight where appropriate.
2. Procedures to ensure that, except as provided in subsection (b) of this section, no boxer is permitted to box while under suspension from any boxing commission due to —
   (A) a recent knockout or series of consecutive losses;
   (B) an injury, requirement for a medical procedure, or physician denial of certification;
   (C) failure of a drug test;
   (D) the use of false aliases, or falsifying, or attempting to falsify, official identification cards or documents; or
   (E) unsportsmanlike conduct or other inappropriate behavior inconsistent with generally accepted methods of competition in a professional boxing match.
3. Procedures to review a suspension where appealed by a boxer, licensee, manager, matchmaker, promoter, or other boxing service provider, including an opportunity for a boxer to present contradictory evidence.
4. Procedures to revoke a suspension where a boxer —
   (A) was suspended under subparagraph (A) or (B) of paragraph (2) of this subsection, and has furnished further proof of a sufficiently improved medical or physical condition; or
   (B) furnishes proof under subparagraph (C) or (D) of paragraph (2) that a suspension was not, or is no longer, merited by the facts.
      (b) Suspension in another state A boxing commission may allow a boxer who is under suspension in any state to participate in a professional boxing match.

1. for any reason other than those listed in subsection (a) of this section if such commission notifies in writing and consults with the designated official of the suspending state's boxing commission before the grant of approval for such individual to participate in that professional boxing match; or
2. if the boxer appeals to the ABC and the ABC determine that the suspension of such boxer was without sufficient grounds, for an improper purpose, or not related to the health and safety of the boxer or the purposes of this article.

### Reporting

Not later than 48 business hours after the conclusion of a professional boxing match, the supervising boxing commission shall report the results of such boxing match and any related suspensions to each boxer.

### Health, safety, and equipment

The Secretary of Health and Human Services shall conduct a study to develop recommendations for health, safety, and equipment standards for boxers and for professional boxing matches.

### Standards and licensing (with respect to boxing matches conducted on Indian Reservations)

If a tribal organization regulates professional boxing matches pursuant to paragraph (1), the tribal organization shall, by tribal ordinance or resolution, establish and provide for the implementation of health and safety standards, licensing requirements, and other requirements relating to the conduct of professional boxing matches that are at least as restrictive as; (1) the otherwise applicable standards and requirements of a State in which the reservation is located; or (2) the most recently published version of the recommended regulatory guidelines certified and published by the Association of Boxing Commissions.

### The Muhammad Ali Boxing Reform Act

In 2000, to further improve and expand the welfare of professional boxers, Congress amended the Federal Boxing Act by enacting the Muhammad Ali Boxing Reform Act (the "Ali Act").[6] The Ali Act was sponsored by Sen. John McCain [R-AZ], Sen. Spencer Abraham [R-MI], Sen. Byron Dorgan [D-ND], Sen. Richard Bryan [D-NV], and Rep. Michael Oxley [R-OH]. Whereas the focus of the Federal Boxing Act was the protection of the boxer *inside* the ring, the Ali Act was enacted primarily for the purpose of protecting the boxer from exploitation *outside* the ring, as well as to promote the overall integrity of the boxing industry. For example, the Ali Act provides for minimum contractual guidelines, prohibition of conflicts of interest between promoters and managers as well as sanctioning bodies, and also contains enforcement provisions, including imprisonment and severe fines for violations of the act.[7] In addition, the Ali Act contains several required disclosures to protect the boxer, including the following disclosure that is relevant to and directly related to the ringside physician's role:

> *HEALTH AND SAFETY DISCLOSURES—It is the sense of the Congress that a boxing commission should, upon issuing an identification card to a boxer under subsection (b) (1), make a health and safety disclosure to that boxer as that commission considers appropriate. The health and safety disclosure should include the health and safety risks associated with boxing, and, in particular, the risk and frequency of brain injury and the advisability that a boxer periodically undergo medical procedures designed to detect brain injury.[8]*

### Additional Legislation

Despite the efforts of Senator John McCain and other members of both the Congress and Senate, many federal bills which, if passed, would have effectively created a national commission for professional boxing have been defeated. A list is given here of some of these bills and the ultimate result of the legislation:[9]

110th Congress: S. 84 *Dead*
110th Congress: H.R. 4031 *Dead*

109th Congress: S. 148 *Passed Senate*
109th Congress: H.R. 468 *Dead*
108th Congress: S. 275 *Passed Senate*
108th Congress: S. 2603 *Passed Senate*
108th Congress: S. 3021 *Passed Senate*
108th Congress: H.R. 1281 *Dead*
107th Congress: S. 2550 *Dead*
107th Congress: H.R. 5006 *Dead*
106th Congress: S. 143: Professional Boxing Safety Act Amendments *Dead*
104th Congress: S. 187 *Passed Senate*
104th Congress: H.R. 1150 *Dead*
104th Congress: H.R. 1186 *Dead*
104th Congress: H.R. 4114 *Dead*
104th Congress: H.R. 4167 *Enacted*
103rd Congress: S. 1991 *Dead*
103rd Congress: H.R. 4753 *Dead*

### Pending Legislation

In 2009, Senator John McCain (R-AZ), with the assistance of Senator Byron Dorgan (D-ND) and Congressman Peter King (R-NY) introduced S38 and H.R. 523, the Professional Boxing Amendments Act of 2009. If enacted, this bill will form the United States Boxing Commission, which will oversee all aspects of professional boxing. Included in the bill are improved medical safety standards that would provide for a medical registry and adoption of uniform infectious disease testing, and would ensure that properly trained medical personnel and a requirement that trained physicians be present at all times during a contest.

### LEGAL

Each physician takes an oath to practice medicine to the best of their ability, to protect and preserve life, do no harm, and exercise ethically and moral behavior while treating a patient. This oath includes caring for athletes in professional sports. Although some will question a physician working in a sport in which the aim is to injure the opponent, most of these critics fail to recognize that intent and outcome are very different in professional boxing. Moreover, though perceived as a dangerous sport, in reality boxing is ranked below football, auto racing, and horse racing in fatalities[10] and below popular sports such as cheerleading, soccer, and gymnastics in frequency of injuries.[11] Regardless, there are legal ramifications for any physician involved in professional sports.

Because of the economic environment in sports in which athletes commonly sign multi-million dollar contracts, doctors, trainers, and other professionals are at risk for being held responsible, or at least being caught up in some litigation, should injuries occur. Unlike the team physician who may be responsible for the medical services to the individual athletes of a team, ringside physicians are usually independent contractors working for a boxing commission. Thus, although these doctors are working for a commission, they may not be working under the auspices of the commission and will therefore be at additional risk should an injury or catastrophe occur. There are several steps a ringside physician may take to minimize their risk:

1. Obtain supplemental malpractice insurance covering sports-related activity:
   Many carriers may be hesitant to issue sports-related malpractice insurance in fear of high liability should a law suit occur. However, the ringside physician should

check with his or her insurance carrier as many will issue this additional rider for a nominal fee or even include it in an existing policy.

2. Include an indemnification clause in the fighter's contract:

Many commissions have included clauses in their fighter contracts to protect the commission and its agents. One can contact one's local commission and request or demand that they include the ringside physician in this language. Although this will not prevent a successful law suit in the instance where negligence occurs, it will certainly decrease the doctor's potential liability and even make it more likely that the insurance carrier will include sports-related activities in an existing policy. The language may include the following example:

*The Unarmed Combatant understands that by participating in the scheduled contest or exhibition, the Unarmed Combatant is engaging in an extremely dangerous activity. The Unarmed Combatant further understands that this participation subjects the Unarmed Combatant to a risk of severe injury or death. The Unarmed Combatant, with full knowledge of the risk, nonetheless, agrees to enter into this agreement and hereby waives any claim that the Unarmed Combatant or Unarmed Combatant's heirs may have against the Commission, its entities and instrumentalities, and, to the maximum extent permitted by applicable law, the attending ringside physicians, as the result of any injury the Unarmed Combatant may suffer as a result of Unarmed Combatant's participation in any contest of boxing. I have read and understand the above. (initial) _____.*

3. Become an agent of the commission:

As a member of an entity, unless gross malpractice occurs, it is unlikely that the physician can be held individually liable for bad outcomes during a contest. Although most ringside physicians operate independently of the commission, it is advisable for the physician to approach the local commission and explore the ways he or she may become an employee or member of the commission. Unfortunately, many ringside physicians are still paid directly by the promoter, thus increasing exposure. To circumvent this obstacle, the ringside physician should have the commission request that the promoter pay this fee to the commission and then have the commission pay the fee to the doctor for services rendered. This action consolidates that the doctor is working as an agent of the commission and reduces liability and exposure. Local jurisdiction should be consulted for rules and regulations pertaining to liability and responsibilities for agents of a commission.

4. Have the commission obtain malpractice insurance for the physician:

The physician inquires whether his or her commission has the ability to secure coverage for one's activity as a ringside physician. In most cases, the cost is much lower for the commission to purchase this coverage and it often contains higher coverage limits.

5. Maintain a medical license for the jurisdiction of the fight

It is important to recognize that malpractice insurance will not necessarily cover the ringside physician who is practicing medicine out of state, where the doctor may not be licensed; similar to a traveling team physician. The physician should check with his or her carrier before working in a jurisdiction not in their locale.

6. Maintain complete documentation

One of the most commons issues in malpractice suits applies to the standard of care. To ensure that the physician maintains accepted practice, it is imperative that all examinations be documented. Each competitor should receive a pre-participation medical requirement form and be required to meet each of these predetermined qualifications before being certified to compete. In addition, the pre-fight examination form, post-fight examination form, and suspension form should be completed by the ringside physician and given to the commission. Furthermore, a copy of the suspension form should be given to the participant along with any additional instructions for post-fight medical care. Finally, all results should be reviewed with the commission. It is obviously imperative to obtain a medical release to satisfy all Health Insurance Portability and Accountability Act regulations before discussing any medical information with the commission or its agents.

In the event that a fighter is prohibited from competing this information must be well documented, as some athletes have sued physicians for this refusal. Nevertheless, if a participant does not pass the pre-fight evaluation, they should never be permitted to compete regardless of the significance of the contest. In addition, the competitor with a pre-existing medical condition must not be allowed to sign a waiver indemnifying the doctor and commission from liability, because this will not completely protect the doctor and is obviously not protecting the health and safety of the competitor.

## SUMMARY

The administration, legislative, ethical, and legal aspects of ringside medicine continue to evolve. As legislation proceeds, the enforcement of rules and regulations will change as well. In the absence of a national commission to oversee professional boxing, it is more imperative for the ringside physician to understand and implement the additional precautions, as well as the unique skills required by ringside medicine to ensure that the health and safety of the athletes are preserved. It is equally important for the doctors to protect their interests to minimize their own liability risks. Over the next few years, a national commission should be created and oversight will improve, ensuring that the professional fighter's interests are properly protected.

## REFERENCES

1. Minimum medical requirements—American Association of Professional Ringside Physicians (2003). Available at: www.aaprp.org.
2. Ethical guidelines—American Association of Professional Ringside Physicians (2005). Available at: www.aaprp.org.
3. Pub. L. No. 104-272, 100 Stat. 3309 (1996) (codified as amended at 15 U.S.C. §§ 6301-6313(2000)).
4. The Federal Boxing Act was sponsored by Rep. John Williams [D-MT], Rep. Michael Oxley [R-OH], and Rep. Thomas Manton [D-NY], H.R. (4167). Available at: www.govtrack.us/congress/bill.xpd?bill=h104-4167.
5. Pub. L. No. 104-272, 100 Stat. 3309 (1996) (codified as amended at 15 U.S.C. §§ 6302 (2000).
6. Muhammad Ali Boxing Reform Act, Pub. L. No. 106-210, 114 Stat. 321 (1999) (codified at 15 U.S.C. §§ 6301-6313(2000)).
7. Muhammad Ali Boxing Reform Act, Pub. L. No. 106–210, §3 (purposes), 114 Stat. 321 (2000).
8. Pub. L. No. 104-272, 100 Stat. 3309 (1996) (codified as amended at 15 U.S.C. §§ 6305 (3) (c) (2002).
9. Available at: http://www.govtrack.us/congress/bill.xpd?bill=h103-4753&;tab=related. Accessed February 1, 2009.
10. Cantu R, editor. Boxing and medicine. Illinois: Human Kinetics; 1995. p. xi-xiii.
11. Burt CW, Overpeck MD. Emergency visits for sports-related injuries. Ann Emerg Med 2001;23:301–8.

# Role of the Ringside Physician and Medical Preparticipation Evaluation of Boxers

Michael Kelly, DO

**KEYWORDS**

• Combat sports • Boxing • Martial arts • Ringside physician
• Ring doctor

Ringside physicians play a dynamic and multifaceted role in combat sports. Ring doctors are entrusted with the acute care of injured athletes, the rendering of instant medical opinions on bout termination, and postbout medical care. Many are familiar with ring doctors entering the ring to evaluate injured fighters, but few realize the extensive preparation and long hours that are required. The work of a ringside physician begins long before the first bout starts and ends long after the last fan has left the arena.

Before each show, designated ringside physicians review each fighter's medical record to ensure that there are no medical conditions that may endanger the welfare of a fighter or their opponent. Most states require periodic blood tests, physical examinations, electrocardiograms, dilated eye exams, and brain scans.

A number of abnormalities are often found on prelicensing medical testing. Meningiomas, porencephaly, encephalomalacia, chronic and acute subdural hematomas, ischemic brain injury, colloid cysts, and even vascular malformations have been found on prelicensing brain imaging. Such findings usually disqualify fighters from participation. CT scanning is a popular choice for pre- and postfight brain imaging because it is readily available and relatively inexpensive when compared to MRI scanning. However, MRI scanning is more sensitive for chronic traumatic brain injury.[1,2] MRI scans of fighters often reveal nonspecific white matter changes. At this time, the clinical implication of these findings is unknown. Progressive white matter changes on serial brain MRI scans usually requires further investigation before a fighter is cleared to compete. This is a valid argument for serial brain imaging in fighters.

Ocular examinations performed on fighters may reveal chronic traumatic injury. Routine dilated ocular examinations submitted to licensing boards have revealed retinal detachment, lattice formation, cornea scaring, early glaucoma, and cataracts. The incidence of ocular injury in fighters was previously believed to be higher in fighters but the risk of ocular injury may be decreasing with stricter medical supervision.[3,4]

Procare Medical Associates, 124 E. Mount Pleasant Avenue, Livingston, NJ 07039, USA
E-mail address: fightmedicine@gmail.com

Clin Sports Med 28 (2009) 515–519
doi:10.1016/j.csm.2009.07.003
sportsmed.theclinics.com
0278-5919/09/$ – see front matter © 2009 Elsevier Inc. All rights reserved.

Cardiovascular incidents are unusual in fighters. However, prebout ECGs and cardiovascular screening may reveal abnormalities such as rhythm disturbances, structural heart disease, and evidence of rare diseases such as prolonged QT interval syndrome. Interpretation of fighter's ECGs is challenging because of the increased incidence of athletic heart syndrome. Furthermore, a recent study suggested that nonspecific ECG changes in the anterior leads may predict future cardiovascular disease.[5–7]

Prebout serology includes testing for anemia, platelet disorders, coagulation disorders, and infectious diseases including HIV and hepatitis. Interpretation of blood counts may be complicated by the development of pseudoanemia and pseudoerythrocytosis. Pseudoanemia occurs when the fighter increases training intensity in a warm environment resulting in plasma expansion and hemodilution. Pseudoerythrocytosis occurs when a fighter dehydrates in an attempt to control weight.[8]

A positive HIV test mandates an indefinite medical suspension. Transmission of a blood borne life-threatening disease can occur. Similarly, an infection with hepatitis B or C may also prevent a fighter from competing. There is at least one documented case of hepatitis C transmission during an altercation.[9]

Occasionally, fighters may have evidence of a disease on the physical exam performed by the fighter's personal physician and submitted to the licensing board. Such situations usually require further workup and risk assessment before competition.

Once fighters have completed the sanctioning state's prefight medical testing they must undergo a physical examination by a ringside physician at the weigh-in or event. The prefight examination begins with questions about the fighter's general health, medications, record, knockouts, injuries, neurological status, and cardiovascular status. The prefight interview also allows the ring doctor to become familiar with the fighter's speech patterns and behavior, which may prove useful when assessing a knockout.

Prefight medical questions may include:

- Do you have any medical problems? If so, please explain.
- Have you seen a doctor for any issues other than routine health?
- Do you take any medications?
- Have you taken any medication or had any injections recently?
- Have you received any joint injections in the past month?
- Do you have any old or recent injuries?
- Do you have any visual disturbances?
- How many fights have you had?
- Have you ever been knocked out? If yes, how many times and when was the last time?
- Have you ever been unconscious for any other reason?
- When you train, do you have any shortness of breath, chest pain, palpitations, or lightheadedness?

A brief physical examination follows the prefight interview. Ringside physicians examine the fighter for injuries or medical conditions that could increase a fighter's risk of injury in the ring. Examples include unhealed lacerations, active skin infections, orthopedic injuries, internal organ injuries, ocular injuries, cardiac abnormalities, pulmonary abnormalities, and neurological abnormalities. The prefight examination places special emphasis on the face, eyes, neck, spine, ribs, and hands. Occasionally, information is obtained that may require bout cancellation but usually information gleaned from the prefight evaluation is used by ring doctors making difficult judgments during bouts.

The prefight evaluation of the head and neck involves careful examination of the skin for unhealed lacerations and infections. It is important to examine the back of the ears for occult lacerations. Palpation of the maxillary, ocular, nasal, and jaw bones may reveal areas of injury. Palpable crepitus with an absence of bruising may indicate a facial fracture nonunion. Examination of the oropharyrnx should include evaluation of the mucosa for dehydration and tooth misalignment indicative of a previous mandible fracture. Careful attention should be directed to the ocular examination. Pupil irregularities should be noted as well as extraocular movements.

The prefight evaluation of the musculoskeletal system is assessed with extra attention on the spine, ribs, and hands. Crepitus or tenderness over the ribcage may indicate a fractured rib and require bout termination. Deformities of the knuckles and wrists are common. Enlarged metacarpophalangeal joints with displacement of the extensor tendon may indicate previous injury of the sagittal bands or capsule. Enlarged nontender knuckles do not disqualify a fighter from competition. Professional fighters may have a history of metacarpal fracture involving the third metacarpal; not the fifth metacarpal as commonly believed. Repetitive injury to the carpometacarpal joint can cause an enlargement of the dorsal aspect of the wrist called bossing. Nontender, subtle wrist deformities with normal function, motion, and strength do not disqualify a fighter from competition.

The prefight evaluation of the cardiovascular system includes auscultation, pulse, and blood pressure, which may reveal bradycardia, tachycardia, relative hypotension, murmurs, and thrills. Bradycardia is a common finding. Blood pressures are usually within normal ranges but tend to be lower in the lighter weights and higher in the heaver weights. Hypotension combined with tachycardia and dry mucus membranes may indicate poor hydration and unsafe weight loss practices. A severely dehydrated fighter may be disqualified from competition. Systolic murmurs can occur in conditioned athletes but any fighter with a diastolic murmur or a systolic murmur that worsens with a valsalva maneuver should be further evaluated before being cleared for competition.

The prefight evaluation of the pulmonary system includes evaluation of the respiratory rate and lung auscultation. Lung sounds should be clear. Irregularities can include wheezing with poorly treated asthma or crackles indicative of active lung infection both of which may require bout termination.

The prefight evaluation of the neurological system begins with an interview and ends with an evaluation of the fighter's speech, memory, concentration, and gait. Slow, slurred speech or abnormal responses may indicate early chronic traumatic brain injury. A broad-based clumsy gait may indicate early motor disease. Reflexes are usually normal and coordination abnormalities may be difficult to access in a professional athlete.

Once an event begins, the ringside physicians monitor the fighters' coordination, agility, and aggressiveness in addition to any obvious injuries. Fighters with concussive brain injury often have subtle changes in coordination, agility, and aggressiveness that can be quickly identified by an observant ringside physician. Ringside physicians may be called upon to render an expert medical opinion concerning bout termination and fighter injury. This responsibility poses a unique challenge because the physician is required to quickly access the injury and determine the immediate prognosis within seconds.

Ringside physicians may recommend bout termination if a fighter is deemed to have a serious injury. Such recommendations are not taken lightly. There are a number of medical issues that may result in bout termination, including lacerations, concussion, ocular injuries, excessive head trauma, and orthopedic injuries. Lacerations involving the eyelid, lacrimal system, or uncontrolled bleeding affecting fighter vision require bout termination.

The decision to recommend bout termination is based on the premise that the ringside physician is present to protect the fighter. Such decisions are complex and require training, experience, medical knowledge, judgment, and ethics. During the heat of the moment, fighters and their seconds may be angry but such emotions are usually short-lived. Most fighters appreciate the fact that ringside physicians are present for their safety.

When a knockout or serious injury occurs, ringside physicians are expected to provide urgent medical care. The primary goal is to ensure safe evacuation of the injured fighter to the nearest trauma center. Every unconscious fighter is assumed to have a cervical spinal cord injury until proven otherwise. The airway and circulation are assessed. The decision to remove a mouthpiece is based on airway obstruction. If it obstructs the airway, it is removed. In the event that a fighter does not regain consciousness within 1 minute, the fighter should be evacuated to the nearest trauma center. The extraction of an injured fighter should not be delegated to emergency medical technicians. The extraction of an injured fighter from a boxing ring poses a unique challenge. The ringside physician should take control of the situation and ensure that the spine is stabilized, oxygen administered, and that the fighter is appropriately logrolled onto a backboard before transport. Fortunately, the majority of fighters quickly regain consciousness.

After a bout, every fighter is evaluated by a ringside physician. There are two goals at this stage. The first is to administer urgent medical care and the second is to order appropriate follow-up testing and medical consultations. The majority of injuries are self-limited but occasionally a fighter may be sent to the hospital for emergency care. Fighters are often pressured into fighting before they are fully healed and, because of this, medical suspensions are ordered by ringside physicians to ensure injured fighters have adequate healing time and appropriate medical care. Such actions are intended to protect the fighter and are not punitive. The length of suspension should correlate with injury severity and medical literature not arbitrary numbers.

Common injuries encountered during the postfight examination include concussive brain injury, facial fractures, lacerations, and hand injuries.

The most concerning is traumatic brain injury. There may be subtle signs of concussion immediately after a bout. Occasionally fighters become more symptomatic with time. Worsening concussive symptoms should raise the suspicion of a traumatic brain injury and the fighter should be sent to the nearest trauma center. The most common cause of fighter death is a subdural hematoma.[10,11] It is important to remember that even bout winners may suffer from traumatic brain injury.

Lacerations are common and may require suture or tissue adhesive repair to ensure adequate healing and maximum wound strength. Large lacerations and those requiring multilayered closure may require a medical suspension to ensure adequate healing time.

Hand and wrist injuries commonly occur and it is important for the ringside physician to examine the unwrapped hands after a bout. The metacarpal and carpal bones should be palpated for crepitus and tenderness. Any suspected fracture requires radiographs and possibly an orthopedic consultation. Swollen knuckles may indicate an intraarticular fracture, tears of the radial sagittal bands, or joint capsule tears. Occasionally, the extensor mechanism is injured.

Ocular injuries occur in boxing. Common postfight findings include ecchymosis, eyelid edema, and injection. Traumatic iritis can cause injection and miosis in the affected eye. Corneal abrasions can occur and are easily seen with fluorescein stain.

Fighters with complaints of visual field deficits or "floaters" should be seen by an ophthalmologist as soon as possible.

It is common for injured fighters to realize the extent of their injuries after the adrenalin rush from a fight has dissipated. Such fighters usually require a repeat assessment. Upon completion of the event, ringside physicians should walk through the dressing rooms and make sure there are no unattended, injured fighters.

Ringside medicine is a unique subspecialty of sports medicine that has a number of unique challenges. The rapid evaluation of injuries and rendering of medical decisions can be difficult but rewarding. Ringside physicians often arrive early and leave late. They juggle multiple responsibilities while trying to provide fair medical judgments and quality medical care. Although such challenges are difficult, they have incredible rewards. After all, the ringside physician has the best seat in the house.

## REFERENCES

1. Le TH, Gean AD. Neuroimaging of traumatic brain injury. Mt Sinai J Med 2009; 76(2):145–62.
2. Manolakaki D, Velmahos GC, Spaniolas K, et al. Early magnetic resonance imaging is unnecessary in patients with traumatic brain injury. J Trauma 2009; 66(4):1008–12.
3. Giovinazzo VJ, Yannuzzi LA, Sorenson JA, et al. The ocular complications of boxing. Ophthalmology 1987;94(6):587–96.
4. Bianco M, Vaiano AS, Colella F, et al. Ocular complications of boxing. Br J Sports Med 2005;39(2):70–4.
5. Pelliccia A, Di Paolo FM, Quattrini FM, et al. Outcomes in athletes with marked ECG repolarization abnormalities. N Engl J Med 2008;358(2):152–61.
6. Hauser AM, Dressendorfer RH, Vos M, et al. Symmetric cardiac enlargement in highly trained endurance athletes: a two-dimensional echocardiographic study. Am Heart J 1985;109(5 Pt 1). p. 1038–44.
7. Urhausen A, Kindermann W. Echocardiographic findings in strength- and endurance-trained athletes. Sports Med 1992;13(4):270–84.
8. Kelly M. Fight medicine, diagnosis and treatment of combat sports injuries for boxing, wrestling, and mixed martial arts. Boulder (CO): Paladin Press; 2008; p. 249–51.
9. Bourliere M, Halfon P, Quentin Y, et al. Covert transmission of hepatitis C virus during bloody fisticuffs. Gastroenterology 2000;119(2):507–11.
10. Jordan BD, Levin HS. Medical aspects of boxing. Boca Raton (FL): CRC Press; 1992. p. 189.
11. Unterharnscheidt F, Unterharnscheidt JT. Boxing medical aspects. San Diego (CA): Academic Press; 2003. p. 274.

# Cardiovascular Issues in Boxing and Contact Sports

Stephen A. Siegel, MD, FACC, FACSM[a,b,*]

KEYWORDS

• Cardiovascular risks • Cardiac evaluation • Boxing
• Cardiac contusion • Coronary heart disease

Despite the inherent traumatic nature of boxing and contact sports, there are relatively few reports of boxing-associated cardiovascular (CV) events. This may be related to the type of force that is applied to the chest with a gloved hand and the anatomy of the heart in the chest. The heart, as opposed to the brain, is mobile and padded in the thoracic cavity and less prone to acceleration-deceleration injuries that routinely occur during a boxing match. The age and general condition of the participants is also different from most recreational athletes. Despite a recent increase in boxing as CV exercise training, the general population is young and well trained. On the other end of the age spectrum, participation in the more vulnerable pre-teen and teenage athlete (such as is present in baseball) is more limited and controlled. The duration of exercise in boxing is limited and although there is evidence of hyper adrenergic activity because of the competition, the period of sustained elevation of heart rate (HR) and blood pressure (BP) are limited. The extensive conditioning necessary for competitive boxing reduces the chances of a subclinical pathology from reaching the competitive arena. Environmental factors are also limited, as boxing is generally performed in a controlled environment, without wide extremes of either temperature or humidity.

Even with these caveats, boxing requires a high level of physical effort that may tax the abilities of an abnormal or susceptible heart. The metabolic demand of 1 hour of boxing is equivalent to running 9 km in 60 minutes on the treadmill.[1] The chest trauma incurred from a blow or fall may damage even this protected vital organ. This article discusses the nature of intrinsic and traumatic CV risk with boxing with a focus on the underlying anatomy and physiology of cardiac, vascular, and arterial damage.

[a] Department of Medicine, Leon H. Charney Division of Cardiology, New York University School of Medicine, 245 East 35th Street, New York, NY 10016, USA
[b] Greater New York Regional Chapter, American College of Sports Medicine, 245 East 35th Street, New York, NY 10016, USA
* Department of Medicine, Leon H. Charney Division of Cardiology, NYU School of Medicine, 245 East 35th Street, New York, NY 10016.
E-mail address: stephen.siegel@nyumc.org

Clin Sports Med 28 (2009) 521–532
doi:10.1016/j.csm.2009.07.001
0278-5919/09/$ – see front matter © 2009 Elsevier Inc. All rights reserved.

## BACKGROUND

The heart sits protected by the rib cage and the thoracic musculature. It is suspended by attachments to the posterior chest wall, however is mobile within the pericardial sac and thorax during normal function. The coronary arteries lie embedded in grooves in the surface of the heart. Fatty tissue is usually present that also reduces the risk of direct injury to the coronary arteries.

Atherosclerotic disease of the coronary arteries may begin in the second decade of life but is usually nonobstructive, only involving the subintimal region of the artery. Most myocardial infarctions (MI) occur because of rupture of the subintimal atherosclerotic plaque and most commonly occur (70%) in arteries that are not severely obstructed (<75%). This may occur at any time, but exercise has been documented to increase the risk of plaque rupture. This occurs less in the well-trained aerobically fit than in sedentary individuals.

Sudden cardiac death (SCD) is generally an arrhythmic event with the development of ventricular tachycardia or other hemodynamically unstable rhythm. Several types of genetic predispositions have been identified, including abnormalities in myocardial membrane channels and anatomic abnormalities of the right ventricle and conduction system.[2] These abnormalities are generally rare, however may become clinically apparent in the second and third decades of life when competitive athletic participation is greatest.

## CARDIOVASCULAR RISKS OF EXERCISE

Cardiovascular events are catastrophic, occurring in otherwise healthy people frequently in the prime of their life and are met with publicity and blame. Because of the relatively low incidence of CV events with exercise, there are widely divergent rates reported in the literature. Among the millions of teenage athletes competing in the United States, approximately 10 to 13 such cases are reported every year.[3] The rates differ by age, gender, and geography, occurring more commonly in older athletes and men. In the older athlete, atherosclerotic disease becomes the predominate risk. Sudden cardiac death or myocardial infarction during exercise is usually associated with rupture of an atherosclerotic plaque with subsequent obstruction of the coronary artery. As competitive boxers are generally younger athletes, we will focus on the risks for those younger than 35 years old.

There are numerous physical and physiologic adaptations by the heart to the demands of chronic intense exercise. These changes, although considered normal variations and not pathologic, are similar to abnormalities that may result in injury. In general, athletes who train with significant resistance loads develop hypertrophy of the left ventricle (LV) with minimal increase in LV volume, whereas prolonged low-resistance training will result in higher LV volume and cardiac output without as large an increase in ventricular mass and thickness. The training required for competitive boxing frequently entails both resistance and prolonged aerobic exercise. The changes that occur may mimic many of the abnormalities discussed and make screening and diagnosis more difficult.

In autopsy studies of death in young athletes, 95% demonstrate a structural abnormality.[4] Inheritable cardiomyopathies and congenital coronary artery anomalies account for most of the events, with valvular heart disease, Marfan syndrome, dilated cardiomyopathy, and myocarditis being the remainder of the myocardial abnormalities and premature coronary atherosclerosis and myocardial bridging affecting the coronary circulation. The remaining 5% of events without a structural anomaly probably represent arrhythmogenic events related to long QT syndrome, Brugada syndrome, cathecholaminergic polymorphic ventricular tachycardia, or noncardiogenic extrinsic factors such as drugs.

Hypertrophic cardiomyopathy (HCM) is the most common cause of SCD in young athletes accounting for more than 30% of the cases. It is an autosomal dominant trait with variable penetration and a prevalence of 0.2%.[2] There are several identified mutations that affect sarcomere proteins. It is a primary disease of cardiac muscle that results in hypertrophy without LV dilation. Several variations exist, however the most common involves the septum out of proportion to the free walls. Microscopically, myocardial disarray is generally seen with diffuse interstitial fibrosis and involvement of the intramural coronary arteries. Symptoms such as dyspnea, chest pain, dizziness, or syncope are variable, affecting only approximately 20% of athletes in one series[4] The electrocardiogram (ECG), however, is more commonly abnormal with 90% demonstrating abnormalities such as left atrial deviation, diffuse symmetric and marked T-wave inversion, ST segment depression, increased voltage in the precordial leads, or deep Q waves[5] The most diagnostic test is an echocardiogram. There is an extensive literature of the types of abnormalities seen in hypertrophic cardiomyopathy but the hallmark is LV hypertrophy. There are several modifying factors that help to distinguish this from the normal enlargement of the LV that occurs with training; however, no definite specific echocardiographic feature has been identified.

Congenital coronary artery anomalies are an infrequent condition affecting 0.1% to 0.2% of the general population; however, it is the most common cause of SCD in young women and the etiology in approximately 20% of all cases of SCD in young athletes.[4] The resting ECG is usually normal and even stress testing may have a limited role in detecting these abnormalities. Transthoracic echocardiography can frequently identify the left main and proximal right coronary artery[6]; however, transesophageal echocardiography has a higher sensitivity and coronary angiography is definitive. Advances in CT angiography and MR angiography provide alternative noninvasive definitive diagnostic tools. Because this is a correctable disease, diagnosis is essential. Exercise-induced chest pain or syncope is the primary warning sign, although they were present in only 30% of athletes who collapsed from congenital coronary artery anomalies.[7]

Myocarditis is an acute or chronic inflammatory process of the myocardium that leads to myocyte dysfunction and development of an arrhythmogenic substrate. It is generally infectious in origin (usually viral) and therefore occurs more commonly in close living conditions such as dormitories or barracks. Symptoms such as exercise intolerance, fatigue, and dyspnea with signs of congestive heart failure (CHF) on examination are significant; especially with the history of a recent viral illness. Myocarditis typically involves patches of myocardium and therefore may result in arrhythmias without the development of cardiac dysfunction or symptoms. If there is evidence of myocarditis, athletes must be withdrawn from training and competition. Assessment of the residual arrhythmogenic potential must be considered before return to exercise.[8]

Dilated cardiomyopathy involves dilation of the left ventricle opposed to LV wall hypertrophy seen in hypertrophic cardiomyopathy. The etiology in younger athletes is commonly viral and may be the later manifestation of myocarditis. In older individuals this may be the result of chronic or recurrent ischemia, hypertension, or diabetes. As opposed to the normal dilation that is seen in many athletes, there is impaired systolic function. Warning signs are similar to myocarditis with symptoms of heart failure; however, the severity can vary and is commonly asymptomatic. Echocardiography is usually necessary for diagnosis and in mild cases can be confused with athlete's heart.[9]

Marfan syndrome is a multisystemic illness that is a genetic disorder of connective tissue with characteristic traits including tall stature, arachnodactyly, hyperextensible joints, pectus excavatum, and scoliosis. The defect results in weakness of the aortic media with cystic medial necrosis.[10] Echocardiography demonstrates dilation of the aortic root and proximal ascending aorta. Mitral valve prolapse is also common. The physiologic stress of competitive athletics with increased BP, HR, and LV contractility may result in aortic dissection or rupture especially with an aortic root larger than 6 cm.[11] The morphologic features common in Marfan (tall and lanky) may limit the likelihood that they will participate in competitive boxing (as opposed to basketball); however, the clinical manifestations vary greatly and even mild physical abnormalities suggestive of Marfan should instigate an echocardiogram.

Valvular disease in the athlete may be congenital or acquired (rheumatic or infectious). Aortic valve stenosis is the most serious valvular abnormality for the athlete as when it is severe it may lead to sudden hemodynamic collapse because of pressure overload of the LV and sudden fall in cardiac output. This is a relatively uncommon cause of CV events and the diagnosis can usually be made by auscultation. The severity of aortic valve stenosis is best determined by echocardiography, and periodic monitoring of less than severe stenosis needs to be monitored to determine progression. Aortic valve regurgitation is a volume overload of the LV, which by itself is generally not associated with sudden collapse. In athletes it may be associated with primary disease of the aortic root with the risk of aortic rupture or dissection. Aortic regurgitation when severe may result in CHF.

Mitral regurgitation is a relatively common valvular abnormality that can result in a volume overload of the left atrium and diastolic volume overload in the left ventricle. When severe it leads to CHF and atrial arrhythmias, especially atrial fibrillation. Mitral valve prolapse (MVP) may result in mitral regurgitation but has been identified as the sole autopsy abnormality is some series. The mechanism of death is not clear and because MVP is extremely common, it may merely be an incidental finding. Mitral stenosis leads to pressure overload of the left atrium and pulmonary hypertension. The left ventricle is generally spared until late in the course but the elevated left atrial and pulmonary artery pressures can lead to dyspnea and CHF. Because the diastolic flow in mitral stenosis is dependent upon heart rate and diastolic filling times, the physiology usually limits the ability to exercise at the high heart rates demanded in training for competitive sports.

Auscultation is frequently adequate to detect valvular disease, although the diastolic murmurs of aortic regurgitation and mitral stenosis may be occult. Echocardiography is usually the definitive diagnostic tool for detection and quantification of valvular disease and is required for assessment of virtually all murmurs.[12]

Detection of undiagnosed complex congenital heart disease in the athlete is rare. The hemodynamic consequences of most of these abnormalities prevent the aerobic capacity necessary to participate; however, in rare circumstances an echocardiogram will detect major abnormalities. Atrial septal defect is commonly not detected until the second decade of life and may lead to the development of left atrial pressure overload, right ventricular failure, CHF, or arrhythmias. Small ventricular septal defects with normal LV size and normal pulmonary pressures are usually not a significant risk of CV events.[13]

Arrhythmias in the absence of identifiable morphologic cardiac abnormalities are usually related to one of several channelopathies. Abnormalities of the ion channel proteins may result in a predisposition to ventricular tachycardia and sudden cardiac death. The types of channel ion abnormalities affect the responsiveness to neuro humoral factors. Some (short QT and Brugada) are exacerbated by vagal stimulation and generally occur during sleep or vagal maneuvers. They are unlikely to result in an exercise-related event; however, the long-QT syndromes are generally catechol-amine-induced arrhythmias, which may be stimulated by the physiologic or psycho-logical stress of competition or vigorous exercise (**Box 1**). Hundreds of genetic mutations have been identified primarily on 10 genes.[14] Most involve three subtypes that code for ventricular repolarization. The most common presentations of the long-QT syndrome are palpitations, presyncope, syncope, and cardiac arrest. The diagnosis may be suggested by a family history of SCD. The key to diagnosis is the re-sting ECG; the upper limits of the QT interval corrected for the heart rate (the QTc) are below 460 msec for women and below 440 msec for men. The Schwartz scoring system[15] has been widely used for diagnosis; however, specific genetic testing is now available for many forms of the disease. Nongenetic causes of long-QT syndrome include numerous medications, medical illnesses, nutritional deficiencies, and head trauma.

Uncommon in the North America but more common in Italy, arrhythmogenic right ventricular dysplasia (ARVD) is characterized by fatty infiltration of the right ventricle with left bundle branch block pattern ventricular tachycardia. Abnormal T waves in the precordium or an epsilon wave (spike in the ST segment in V1-2), can be present on the resting ECG. Echocardiography may demonstrate RV dilation or dysfunction and cardiac MRI may be diagnostic in demonstrating fatty infiltration of the myocardium.[2]

Reentrant supraventricular arrhythmias are a rare cause of serious cardiac events in the trained athlete. The heart rates that occur with these arrhythmias are generally well tolerated and not likely to induce complications. The exception is A-V node bypass syndromes (such as Wolf Parkinson White) where ventricular rates can be excessive, especially in the presence of atrial fibrillation. The presence of an anomalous bypass tract on the ECG should lead athletes to be screened for the possibility of atrial fibril-lation. Radio frequency catheter ablation of the anomalous tract is routine and may allow the athlete to return to competition.

## SPECIFIC RISKS OF BOXING

As opposed to many other sports where trauma is an unintentional occurrence, in boxing it is the goal. The sport has evolved to attempt to limit the long-term conse-quences of the trauma, however some inherent risks remain. These risks may also be present in recreational boxers where deliberate trauma is reduced.

Trauma to the chest can result in cardiac contusion or concussion (commotio cor-dis). Cardiac contusion is the result of forceful trauma to the chest that results in cardiac injury. Most typical of major injuries such as automobile accidents, markers of cardiac injury include enzymes and ECGs are abnormal. The energy required to inflict an injury to the heart through the adult chest wall is generally beyond that in-flicted by even the most forceful gloved punch. In a study by Bianco and colleagues,[16] ECG abnormalities were detected in a significant number of boxers after competition; however, no athlete had clinical or humoral evidence of myocardial damage. They postulated that the ECG abnormalities may be related to sympathetic hyperactivity related to the event.

Commotio cordis resulting in sudden death has been reported in recreational sports including boxing (**Fig. 1**). This cause of sudden death is thought to be related to a blow striking the chest over the heart resulting in an arrhythmia. It requires the blow to occur just before the T wave peak when the heart is most vulnerable to repolarization injury. It is most common in youthful athletes when the chest wall is more deformable.

| **Box 1** |
| **Causes of the Long QT Syndrome (LQTS)** |

*Inherited*

Romano-Ward (autosomal dominant, normal hearing)

Jervell and Lange Nielson (autosomal recessive, sensorineural hearing loss)

LQTS with syndactyly

*Sporadic Acquired*

Drugs

    Antiarrhythmics

        Class IA

            Quinidine

            Procainamide

            Disopyramide

        Class III

            Sotalol

            Dofetilide

            Bretylium

            Amiodarone (rare)

    Antidepressants

        Tricyclics (eg, amitriptyline)

        Tetracyclics

    Antifungals

        Itraconazole

        Ketoconazole

    Antihistamines

        Astemizole

        Terfenadine

    Antimicrobials

        Erythromycin

        Quinolones

        Chloroquine

    Neuroleptics

        Phenothiazines

        Haloperidol

    Organophosphate insecticides

    Promotility agents (cisapride)

Electrolyte derangement

    Hypocalcemia

    Hypokalemia

    Hypomagnesemia

*Medical conditions*

Cardiac

    Myocarditis

    Tumors

Neurologic

    Cerebrovascular accident

    Encephalitis

    Head trauma

    Subarachnoid hemorrhage

Endocrine

    Hypothyroidism

    Pheochromocytoma

Nutritional

    Alcoholism

    Anorexia nervosa

    Liquid-protein diet

    Starvation

*Data from* Basilico FC. Cardiovascular disease in athletes. Am J Sports Med 1999;27(1): 108–21.

Commotio is more common with projectiles, particularly solid core projectiles such as a baseball or hockey puck. The boxing events described by Maron and colleagues[17] involved two bare-fisted adolescents and occurred during a "playful" shadow-boxing match with a jab or push to the chest.

There are no reported episodes of commotio cordis with sanctioned boxing matches. This may be related to the ability of boxing gloves to diffuse the energy of impact to the chest. Commotio cordis requires deformation of the chest wall that may be prevented by some types of chest protectors. One could consider the padding of the gloves to be equivalent to the suggested chest protectors in sports with hard projectiles (eg, baseball, hockey). Subclinical myocardial contusion may be more common than reported because of the absence of symptoms. The 1992 case report by Bellotti and colleagues[18] describes a myocardial contusion in a professional boxer detected several days after the fight during a preoperative evaluation for a detached retina. The patient had no symptoms or physical manifestations of myocardial contusion but abnormalities were present on the ECG and confirmed by enzyme measurements.

Rupture of the aorta has been reported with chest trauma, but as in commotio cordis, the force impacted on the chest may be blunted by padding of gloves. The force of a fall is not sufficient to cause trauma to the normal aorta. The potential for injury is increased in athletes with disease of the aorta including Marfan syndrome and cystic medial necrosis; however, the typical body habitus in these individuals is not conducive to competitive boxing.

Chronic chylous pericardium, presumably from repeated hemopericardium, was reported in one retired professional boxer.[19] The repeated trauma to the chest wall was the only apparent etiology after extensive evaluation. It should be noted that this

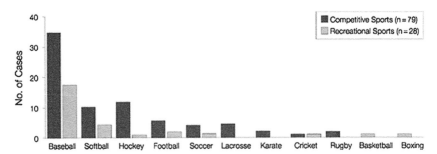

**Fig. 1.** Sports participated in at the time of commotio cordis events. (*From* Maron BJ, Gohman TE, Kyle SB, et al. Clinical profile and spectrum of commotio cordis. JAMA 2002;287(9):1142–6; with permission.)

occurred with lightweight gloves (8 oz) that are no longer used. The improved padding presumably reduces the likelihood of pericardial injury.

## CARDIOVASCULAR EVALUATION OF THE ATHLETE

Routine preparticipation screening of young athletes is recommended by the American Heart Association (AHA) and American College of Sports Medicine (ACSM). It should be noted that these recommendations are based on the consensus of a group of experts in the field and not substantive prospective research.[20] In a joint statement,[21] most recently published in 2007 by both organizations, the guidelines for evaluation are established. The examination should include a detailed personal and family history and a careful physical examination that is directed to detecting the conditions that are associated with exercise-related events. The current American recommendations do not include the routine use of ECGs, which is different from the recommendations of the Europeans. The Study Group on Sports Cardiology of the European Society of Cardiology has adopted the more stringent Italian model for preparticipation screening. The primary difference is the requirement of a 12-lead ECG in addition to a medical history and physical examination.[22] This remains a controversial recommendation with evidence by the Italians that there has been a substantial reduction in mortality because of the detection of cardiomyopathies.[23] However, rebuttal by American experts[20,24] raises several criticisms of expanding the Italian model without further evidence of benefit.

Routine ECG has been advocated to screen for hypertrophic cardiomyopathies; however, the risk of electrophysiologic events may also be reduced by routine ECG screening. In a British-based study of 3500 elite athletes, there was no significant benefit to detecting hypertrophic cardiomyopathies but an unanticipated finding of 15 individuals with either Wolf Parkinson White (WPW) ECG pattern or a long QT interval. Three of nine athletes with long QT were excluded from competitive sports and the six athletes with WPW ECG had an identifiable accessory pathway that was ablated and allowed resumption of competition.[25] Genetic testing of asymptomatic athletes might allow for greatly enhancing the diagnosis of inherited arrhythmogenic cardiomyopathies. Neither the American nor European guidelines include any molecular testing as part of routine guidelines except when there is suspicion of a predisposing problem such as Marfan or long-QT syndrome.[26] The protection of personal genetic information, especially in celebrity athletes, remains a further unresolved issue.

The most consistent reason to exclude further diagnostic tests is the high costs involved with screening the large numbers of potential athletes and the relatively low incidence of abnormalities found. The intensity of the evaluation has to be based on the potential of finding pathology and the risk to the athlete if not detected. The reason for screening is to detect athletes with a potential for unacceptable cardiovascular risk during athletic activities. In addition to the controversy regarding screening, there are also differences with criteria for excluding athletes from participation. There are substantial differences in recommendations between Bethesda #36[27] and the European Society of Cardiology[28] recommendations (**Table 1**).

There are also cultural differences with legal cases in the United States that tested the rights of academic sports programs to exclude athletes based on medical studies

**Table 1**
Summary of selected differences between Bethesda Conference #36 and European Society of Cardiology recommendations for competitive athletes with selected cardiovascular abnormalities

| | Clinical Criteria and Sports Permitted | |
| | BC#36 | ESC |
| --- | --- | --- |
| Gene carriers without phenotype (HCM, ARVC, DCM, ion channel diseases[a]) | All sports | Only recreational sports |
| LQTS | >0.47 s in male subjects, >0.48 s in female subjects<br>Low-intensity competitive sports | >0.44 s in male subjects, >0.46 s in female subjects<br>Only recreational sports |
| Marfan syndrome | If aortic root <40 mm, no MR, no familial SD, then low-moderate intensity competitive sports permitted | Only recreational sports |
| Asymptomatic WPW | EPS not mandatory<br>All competitive sports (restriction for sports in dangerous environment)[a] | EPS mandatory<br>All competitive sports (restriction for sports in dangerous environment)[b] |
| Premature ventricular complexes | All competitive sports, when no increase in PVCs or symptoms occur with exercise | All competitive sports, when no increase in PVCs, couplets, or symptoms occur with exercise |
| Nonsustained ventricular tachycardia | If no CV disease, all competitive sports<br>If CV disease, only low-intensity competitive sports | If no CV disease, all competitive sports<br>If CV disease, only recreational sports |

Abbreviations: ARVC, arrhythmogenic right ventricular cardiomyopathy; BC#36, Bethesda Conference #36; CV, cardiovascular; DCM, dilated cardiomyopathy; EPS, electrophysiologic study; ESC, European Society of Cardiology; HCM, hypertrophic cardiomyopathy; LQTS, long-QT syndrome; MR, magnetic resonance; PVC, premature ventricular complex; SD, sudden death; WPW, Wolff-Parkinson-White syndrome.
[a] Long-QT syndrome, Brugada syndrome, catecholaminergic polymorphic ventricular tachycardia.
[b] Sports in dangerous environments are restricted, given the risk should impaired consciousness occur, such as motor sports, rock climbing, and downhill skiing.
From Pelliccia A, Zipes DP, Maron BJ. Bethesda Conference #36 and the European Society of Cardiology Consensus recommendations revisited. A comparison of US and European criteria for eligibility and disqualification of competitive athletes with cardiovascular abnormalities. J Am Coll Cardiol 2008;52(24):1990–6; with permission.

of risk. At the present time, the courts have upheld the rights of a university-based sports program to exclude an athlete.[29] This has not been definitively expanded to professional sports, however the US Supreme Court held that "the enhanced risk of significant harm to personal health is a legitimate ground for exclusion from employment."[29] It is notorious for athletes with questionable exclusionary diagnosis to "shop" for a physician willing to support their athletic activities. This is especially an issue in the individual activities of a boxer as opposed to a team member where the team owner may be responsible for a deleterious outcome.

Until this is further elucidated, it remains the responsibility of the sports physician to determine whether additional testing is of benefit to the athlete. The potential for liability remains an issue, however knowledge of and adherence to the AHA/ACSM guidelines remains a strong basis for defense.

## DIAGNOSIS AND TREATMENT OF CARDIOVASCULAR EVENTS

The sudden collapse of an athlete is generally related to hemodynamic insufficiency that is benign and merely requires the restoration of adequate volume whether by positional change (Trandelenberg position) or intravenous fluids. In the boxer who develops sudden loss of consciousness regardless of obvious head trauma, cardiovascular collapse must be considered rapidly. The absence of palpable pulse, with or without respirations, must be the trigger to rapidly evaluate and treat an arrhythmia. In the rare episode when there is evidence of a cardiac emergency, the death rate may be reduced by the proper education and preparation of personnel. It has been recommended by the AHA that training in cardiopulmonary resuscitation be routine for trainers and coaches.[30] Automatic External Defibrillators (AEDs) have been encouraged at all fitness facilities by both the AHA and ACSM.[31] This would include competitive events. These simple devices are essential for the potential reversal of a life-threatening arrhythmia but must be urgently used if they are to be effective.

## SUMMARY

Despite the inherent risks associated with exercise in general and boxing in particular, the sport has had a limited number of catastrophic cardiovascular events. Screening should be based on risks involved and become more extensive with the advancement of the athlete. Anatomic and electrophysiologic risks need to be assessed and may preclude participation with resultant life style and economic complications. There should be adequate preparation for the rare potential cardiovascular complication at all events, with the ability to rapidly assess and treat arrhythmias.

## REFERENCES

1. Bellinger B, St Clair Gibson A, Oelofse A, et al. Energy expenditure of a noncontact boxing training session compared with submaximal treadmill running. Med Sci Sports Exerc 1997;29(12):1653–6.
2. Pigozzi F, Rizzo M. Sudden death in competitive athletes. Clin Sports Med 2008; 27(1):153–81.
3. Van Camp S, Bloor C, Mueller F, et al. Nontraumatic sports death in high school and college athletes. Med Sci Sports Exerc 1995;27:641–7.
4. Maron BJ, Shirani J, Polia LC, et al. Sudden death in young competitive athletes. Clinical, demographic and pathological profiles. JAMA 1996;276: 199–204.

5. Maron BJ, Wolfoson JK, Cirò E, et al. Relation of electrocardiographic abnormalities and patterns of left ventricular hypertrophy identified by 2-dimensional echocardiography in patients with hypertrophic cardiomyopathy. Am J Cardiol 1983; 51:189–94.

6. Pelliccia A, Spataro A, Maron BJ. Prospective echocardiographic screening for coronary artery anomalies in 1360 elite competitive athletes. Am J Cardiol 1993;72:978–9.

7. Corrado D, Basso C, Schiavon M, et al. Screening for hypertrophic cardiomyopathy in young athletes. N Engl J Med 1998;339:364–9.

8. Koester MC. A review of sudden cardiac death in young athletes and strategies for preparticipation screening. J Athl Train 2001;36(2):197–204.

9. Pelliccia A, Maron BJ, Spataro A. The upper limit of physiologic cardiac hypertrophy in highly trained athletes. N Engl J Med 1991;324:295–301.

10. Dingemans KP, Teeling P, Van der Wal AC, et al. Ultrastructural pathology of aortic dissections in patients with Marfan syndrome: comparison with dissections in patients without Marfan syndrome. Cardiovasc Pathol 2006;15(4):203–12.

11. Graham TP Jr, Bricker JT, James FW, et al. 26th Bethesda conference: recommendations for determining eligibility for competition in athletes with cardiovascular abnormalities. Task force 1: congenital heart disease. J Am Coll Cardiol 1994;24(4):867–73.

12. Cheitlin MD, Douglas PS, Parmley WW. 26th Bethesda conference: recommendations for determining eligibility for competition in athletes with cardiovascular abnormalities. Task Force 2: Acquired valvular heart disease. J Am Coll Cardiol 1994;24:874–80.

13. Graham TP Jr, Bricker JT, James FW, et al. Task force 1: congenital heart disease. In: Maron BJ, Mitchell JH, editors. 26th Bethesda conference. Recommendations for determining eligibility for competition in athletes with cardiovascular abnormalities. J Am Coll Cardiol 1994;24:867–73.

14. Roden DM. Clinical practice: long QT syndrome. N Engl J Med 2008;358(2): 169–76.

15. Schwartz PJ, Moss AJ, Vincent GM, et al. Diagnostic criteria for the long QT syndrome: an update. Circulation 1993;88:782–4.

16. Bianco M, Colella F, Pannozzo A, et al. Boxing and "commotio cordis": ECG and humoral study. Int J Sports Med 2005;26:151–7.

17. Maron BJ, Gohman TE, Kyle SB, et al. Clinical profile and spectrum of commotio cordis. JAMA 2002;287(9):1142–6.

18. Bellotti P, Chiarella F, Domenicucci S, et al. Myocardial contusion after a professional boxing match. Am J Cardiol 1992;69(6):709–10.

19. Ooi A, Douds AC, Kumar EB, et al. Boxer's pericardium. Eur J Cardiothorac Surg 2003;24:1043–5.

20. Douglas PS. Saving athletes' lives: a reason to find common ground? J Am Coll Cardiol 2008;52(24):1997–9.

21. Maron B, Thompson PD, Ackerman MJ, et al. Recommendations and considerations related to preparticipation screening for cardiovascular abnormalities in competitive athletes: 2007 Update. 2007;115:1643–55.

22. Corrado D, Basso C, Schiavon M, et al. Pre-participation screening of young competitive athletes for prevention of sudden cardiac death. J Am Coll Cardiol 2008;52:1981–9.

23. Corrado D. Trends in sudden cardiovascular death in young competitive athletes after implementation of a preparticipation screening program. JAMA 2006;296: 1593–601.

24. Thompson PD, Levine BD. Protecting athletes from sudden cardiac death. JAMA 2006;296:1648–50.
25. Basavarajaiah S, Wilson M, Whyte G, et al. Prevalence of hypertrophic cardiomyopathy in highly trained athletes: relevance to pre-participation screening. J Am Coll Cardiol 2008;51(10):1033–9.
26. Pelliccia A, Zipes DP, Maron BJ. Bethesda Conference #36 and the European Society of Cardiology Consensus recommendations revisited a comparison of U.S. and European criteria for eligibility and disqualification of competitive athletes with cardiovascular abnormalities. J Am Coll Cardiol 2008;52(24): 1990–6.
27. Maron BJ, Zipes DP. 36th Bethesda Conference: eligibility recommendations for competitive athletes with cardiovascular abnormalities. J Am Coll Cardiol 2005; 45:2–64.
28. Pelliccia A, Fagard R, Bjørnstad HH, et al. Recommendations for competitive sports participation in Athletes with cardiovascular disease: a consensus document from the Study Group of Sports Cardiology of the Working Group of Cardiac Rehabilitation and Exercise Physiology, and the Working Group of Myocardial and Pericardial Diseases of the European Society of Cardiology. Eur Heart J 2005;26:1422–45.
29. Mitten MJ, Maron BJ, Zipes DP. Task Force 12: legal aspects of the 36th Bethesda Conference recommendations. J Am Coll Cardiol 2005;45(8):1373–5.
30. Maron BJ, Thompson PD, Puffer JC, et al. Cardiovascular preparticipation screening of competitive athletes: a statement for health professionals from the Sudden Death Committee (Clinical Cardiology) and Congenital Cardiac Defects Committee (Cardiovascular Disease in the Young), American Heart Association. Circulation 1996;94:850–6.
31. Balady GJ, Chaitman B, Foster C, et al. American Heart Association and American College of Sports Medicine. Automated external defibrillators in health/fitness facilities: supplement to the AHA/ACSM Recommendations for cardiovascular screening, staffing, and emergency policies at health/fitness facilities. Circulation 2002;105:1147–50.

# The Status of Doping and Drug Use and the Implications for Boxing

Gary I. Wadler, MD, FACP, FACSM[a,b,*]

**KEYWORDS**

• Doping • Prohibited list • Therapeutic exemptions • Steroids

*There is no argument that drugs pose at least as serious a health problem in major league sports as they do in most high schools. By the time they have made the pros, most athletes have been given so many pills, salves, injections, potions, by amateur and pro coaches, doctors and trainers, to pick them up, cool them down, kill pain, enhance performance, reduce inflammation, and erase anxiety, that there isn't much they won't sniff, spread, stick in or swallow to get bigger or smaller, or to feel goooood.[1]*

Boxers are not immune from the abuse of drugs.

## HISTORY

History indicates that long ago athletes sought a competitive advantage by using various substances which have been dubbed "ergogenic aids." The third century witnessed the Greeks ingest mushrooms to improve athletic performances; gladiators used stimulants in the famed Circus Maximus (circa 600 BC) to overcome fatigue and injury. By the nineteenth century, athletes experimented with caffeine, alcohol, nitroglycerine, opium, and strychnine.

The first death attributed to doping occurred in 1896 when a Welsh cyclist, Andrew Linton, overdosed on a stimulant, trimethyl, although there is some uncertainty as to the factual basis of this attribution.[2] Nonetheless, there is little doubt that some cyclists died from the use of stimulants in the late nineteenth and early twentieth centuries. Despite these deaths, there was little action taken to address this issue until the death in 1960 of the Dane Knud Jensen during a road race at the Rome Olympic Games. It was not until 1967, the same year still another cyclist, Tommy Simpson at age 29, died of amphetamine use during the Tour de France, that the Union Cycliste

[a] Department of Medicine, NYU School of Medicine, 800 Community Drive, Manhasset, NY 11030, USA
[b] Prohibited List and Methods Committee, World Anti-Doping Agency (WADA), 800 Place Victoria, Suite 1700, PO Box 120, Montreal, QC H4Z 187 Canada
* Department of Medicine, NYU School of Medicine, 800 Community Drive, Manhasset, NY 11030.
E-mail address: wosportgiw@aol.com

Clin Sports Med 28 (2009) 533–543
doi:10.1016/j.csm.2009.06.005
0278-5919/09/$ – see front matter © 2009 Elsevier Inc. All rights reserved.

sportsmed.theclinics.com

International (UC) began to develop a set of rules, and the International Olympic Committee (IOC) created a Medical Commission to combat the misuse of drugs in Olympic Sports.[3] The IOC Medical Commission published the first list of banned drugs for the 1968 Winter Olympics, and in the summer of 1972, at the Munich Olympic Games, drug testing was introduced at an international event. By 1976 the Montreal Olympic Games, the methodology for detecting anabolic steroids in the urine was sufficiently developed to be used in a drug screening program. In the 1983 Pan American Games 19 athletes were disqualified for failed drug tests, 7 of whom were disqualified for anabolic steroid use, and many other athletes withdrew from competition, presumably over concerns about being drug-tested and its potential impact on their Olympic eligibility. However, it was the stripping of the gold medal from the Canadian sprinter Ben Johnson at the 1988 Seoul Olympic Games for doping with the anabolic steroid stanozolol that brought the problem of doping in sports to the attention of the world.

Yet once again it was doping in cycling that changed the perception of the problem of doping in sport. Specifically, in July 1998 a car belonging to team Festina and being driven by the team's soigneur Willy Voet was stopped by customs officers at the French-Belgian border. His car was found to contain an arsenal of more than 400 doping products, including erythropoietin (EPO), stunning the sports world, and leaving a dark shadow hanging over the world's biggest bicycle race. This seminal event led to a paradigm shift in the international community's approach to addressing the abuse of drugs in sports and the eventual establishment of the independent international agency, the World Anti-Doping Agency (WADA) in 1999.

That very same year, 1998, another seminal event occurred in the history of doping when a jar of androstenedione was discovered in the locker of St. Louis Cardinals hitter Mark McGwire who, along with Sammy Sosa, was in pursuit of Roger Maris' all-time baseball record of 61 home runs hit during the 1961 season. McGwire, who admitted to using the testosterone precursor, went on to hit a then record 70 home runs. Baseball subsequently implemented Survey Testing in 2003, with more than 5% of players testing positive for steroids, which set in motion mandatory testing for performance-enhancing drugs for the first time in Major League Baseball (MLB) history. It was in this time frame that the whole BALCO (Bay Area Laboratory Cooperative) affair came to light including the use of the illegal designer steroid, tetrahydrogestinone (THG), leading to the passage of the Anabolic Steroid Control Act that added anabolic steroid precursors, such as androstenedione, to the Schedule III controlled substances.[4]

As sports news became increasingly dominated by stories of doping, the US Congress felt compelled to explore the use of drugs in professional sports leagues that led to the famed hearings before the House Government Reform Committee. Specifically these hearings concerned themselves with doping in MLB and in the National Football League (NFL), and led to significant reforms of the anti-doping policies of both leagues, especially baseball.

In 2006, the book *Game of Shadows*[5] was released detailing the clandestine business of BALCO, a nutritional supplement company that was supplying world-class elite athletes in an array of sports with anabolic steroids, human growth hormone, insulin, EPO, and other performance-enhancing drugs. The book detailed how a self-proclaimed nutritionist and founder of BALCO, Victor Conte, worked with dozens of elite athletes concocting potent cocktails of these drugs to enhance performance. In October 2005, Victor Conte negotiated a plea with federal prosecutors was sentenced to 4 months in federal prison and 4 months of home confinement.

Professional boxing did not escape the taint of the long arm of doping and the shadows of BALCO have cast a cloud over the 2003 match between Oscar De La Hoya and Shane Mosley. Amongst those testifying in 2003 before the BALCO grand jury were track and field athletes Marion Jones, Kevin Toth, Regina Jacobs, Chryste Gaines, and Tim Montgomery; baseball players Barry Bonds, Jason Giambi, Gary Sheffield, and Benito Santiago; football player Bill Romanowski; swimmer Amy Van Dyken; and boxer Shane Mosley.

*In sworn testimony, Mosley himself admits to doping, telling a federal prosecutor that he injected himself with erythropoietin to boost his endurance. He also admitted that he applied a topical cream that contained steroids, as well as using a designer steroid THG, which he indicated he knew was not flaxseed oil.*[6]

Mosley has insisted that he did not know the drugs he took were illegal and filed a defamation lawsuit against Victor Conte, who said he watched Mosley knowingly inject himself with EPO.[7] This match will take place in the courts.

## WORLD ANTI-DOPING AGENCY

Doping not only threatens the health of the athlete whether amateur or professional, it also threatens the integrity of sport and is contrary to the spirit of sport. Before the creation of the WADA, the fight against doping was principally left to individual sports organizations and sport governing bodies. History indicates that these efforts to combat doping, no matter how well intentioned, were not up to the task.

WADA was established in 1999 to promote, coordinate, and monitor the fight against doping in sport in all its forms. Composed and funded equally by the sports movement and governments of the world, WADA coordinated the development and implementation of the World Anti-Doping Code (Code),[8] the document harmonizing anti-doping policies.

For any sports organization to comply with the World Anti-Doping Code it must be sure that their own rules and policies are in compliance with the mandatory articles and other principles of the Code. Athletes in professional sports leagues and organizations that are outside the Olympic movement must comply with the Code when they participate in events or tournaments that are under the jurisdiction of an organization that has implemented the Code, for example, National Basketball Association or NHL players participating in the Olympic Games.[7]

A major strength of WADA is that it is deeply rooted in science, with experts representing a broad array of disciplines including sports medicine, pharmacologists, physiologists, pharmacists, geneticists, and laboratory scientists. Under the umbrella of its Health, Medical & Research Committee, there is the Prohibited List and Methods Committee, Therapeutic Use Exemption Committee, Laboratory Committee, as well as a Gene Doping Panel. These committees meet regularly to assure that WADA's programs and policies remain consistent with the emerging science and other events in the field.

At the core of anti-doping is the list of substances and methods that are prohibited either In- and Out-of-competition or In-competition only. The Prohibited List and Methods Committee meets three times per year to review the List in detail and to recommend any modifications. The proposed changes are reviewed by the stakeholders throughout the world—sports organizations and governments—before being adopted as the Prohibited List in January of the ensuing year.

## DEFINITION OF DOPING

Doping is defined by WADA as the occurrence of one or more of the following anti-doping rule violations:[8]

- Presence of Prohibited Substance:
  Presence of a prohibited substance or its metabolites in an athlete's sample

- Use of Prohibited Substance/Method:
  Use or attempted use by an athlete of a prohibited substance of method
- Refusing Sample Collection:
  Refusing or failing without compelling justification to submit a sample collection after notification as authorized in applicable anti-doping rules, or otherwise evading sample collection
- Failure to File Whereabouts and Missed Tests:
  Violation of applicable requirements regarding athlete availability for out-of-competition testing, including failure to file required whereabouts information and missed test (ie, any combination of three missed tests and/or filing failure within an 18-month period may be deemed a doping violation)
- Tampering:
  Tampering or attempted tampering with any part of the doping control process
- Possession:
  Possession of a prohibited substance and prohibited method
- Trafficking:
  Trafficking or attempted trafficking in any prohibited substance or method
- Administration:
  Administration or attempted administration to an athlete of a prohibited substance and/or method; of assisting, encouraging, aiding, abetting, covering up or any other type of complicity involving an anti-doping rule violation or any attempted anti-doping rule violation.

## STRICT LIABILITY

Under the Code, athletes are strictly liable for the substances found in his or her bodily specimen, and that an anti-doping rule violation occurs whenever a prohibited substance (or its metabolites of markers) is found in bodily specimen, whether or not the athlete intentionally or unintentionally used a prohibited substance or was negligent or otherwise at fault. (WADA Q&A)[8]

## THE 2009 PROHIBITED LIST WORLD ANTI-DOPING CODE

The 2009 Prohibited List World Anti-Doping Code (Adopted from the WADA 2009 Prohibited List)[9]
    The use of any drug should be limited to medically justified indications.
    (All *Prohibited Substances* shall be considered as "Specified Substances" except Substances in classes S1, S2, S.4.4, and S6.a, and *Prohibited Methods* M1, M2, and M3.)
    Where an athlete can establish how a "Specified Substance" entered his or her body or came into his or her possession and that such substance was not intended to enhance the athlete's sports performance or mask the use of a performance-enhancing substance, the Code provides for the elimination or reduction of the period of ineligibility. (WADA Specified Substances)

## SUBSTANCES AND METHODS PROHIBITED AT ALL TIMES (IN- AND OUT-OF-COMPETITION)
### *Prohibited Substances*

---

### *S1. Anabolic agents*
Anabolic agents are prohibited.

1. Anabolic androgenic steroids (AAS)
   a. Exogenous[c] AAS, including:
      **1-androstendiol** (5α-androst-1-ene-3β,17β-diol); **1-androstendione** (5α-androst-1-ene-3,17-dione); **bolandiol** (19-norandrostenediol); **bolasterone; boldenone; boldione** (androsta-1,4-diene-3,17-dione); **calusterone; clostebol; danazol** (17α-ethynyl-17β-hydroxyandrost-4-eno[2,3-d]isoxazole); **dehydrochlormethyltestosterone** (4-chloro-17β-hydroxy-17α-methylandrosta-1,4-dien-3-one); **desoxymethyltestosterone** (17α-methyl-5α-androst-2-en-17β-ol); **drostanolone; ethylestrenol** (19-nor-17α-pregn-4-en-17-ol); **fluoxymesterone; formebolone; furazabol** (17β-hydroxy-17α-methyl-5α-androstano[2,3-c]-furazan); **gestrinone; 4-hydroxytestosterone** (4,17β-dihydroxyandrost-4-en-3-one); **mestanolone; mesterolone; metenolone; methandienone** (17β-hydroxy-17α-methylandrosta-1,4-dien-3-one); **methandriol; methasterone** (2α,17α-dimethyl-5α-androstane-3-one-17β-ol); **methyldienolone** (17β-hydroxy-17α-methylestra-4,9-dien-3-one); **methyl-1-testosterone** (17β-hydroxy-17α-methyl-5α-androst-1-en-3-one); **methylnortestosterone** (17β-hydroxy-17α-methylestr-4-en-3-one); **methyltrienolone** (17β-hydroxy-17α-methylestra-4,9,11-trien-3-one); **methyltestosterone; mibolerone; nandrolone; 19-norandrostenedione** (estr-4-ene-3,17-dione); **norboletone; norclostebol; norethandrolone; oxabolone; oxandrolone; oxymesterone; oxymetholone; prostanozol** (17β-hydroxy-5α-androstano[3,2-c] pyrazole); **quinbolone; stanozolol; stenbolone; 1-testosterone** (17β-hydroxy-5α-androst-1-en-3-one); **tetrahydrogestrinone** (18a-homo-pregna-4,9,11-trien-17β-ol-3-one); **trenbolone** and other substances with a similar chemical structure or similar biologic effect(s).
   b. Endogenous[d] AAS when administered exogenously:
      **androstenediol** (androst-5-ene-3β,17β-diol); **androstenedione** (androst-4-ene-3,17-dione); **dihydrotestosterone** (17β-hydroxy-5α-androstan-3-one); **prasterone** (dehydroepiandrosterone, DHEA); **testosterone** and the following metabolites and isomers: **5α-androstane-3α,17α-diol; 5α-androstane-3α,17β-diol; 5α-androstane-3β,17α-diol; 5α-androstane-3β,17β-diol; androst-4-ene-3α,17α-diol; androst-4-ene-3α,17β-diol; androst-4-ene-3β,17α-diol; androst-5-ene-3α,17α-diol; androst-5-ene-3α,17β-diol; androst-5-ene-3β,17α-diol; 4-androstenediol** (androst-4-ene-3β,17β-diol); **5-androstenedione** (androst-5-ene-3,17-dione); **epi-dihydrotestosterone; epitestosterone; 3α-hydroxy-5α-androstan-17-one; 3β-hydroxy-5α-androstan-17-one; 19-norandrosterone; 19-noretiocholanolone.**
2. Other anabolic agents, including but not limited to:
   Clenbuterol, selective androgen receptor modulators (SARMs), tibolone, zeranol, zilpaterol.

### *S2. Hormones and related substances*
The following substances and their releasing factors are prohibited:

1. **Erythropoiesis-stimulating agents** (eg, **erythropoietin** [EPO], **darbepoietin** [dEPO], **hematide**);

---

[c] "Exogenous" refers to a substance that is not ordinarily capable of being produced by the body naturally.

[d] "Endogenous" refers to a substance that is capable of being produced by the body naturally.

2. **Growth hormone** (GH), **insulin-like growth factors** (eg, IGF-1), **mechano growth factors** (MGFs);
3. **Chorionic gonadotrophin** (CG) and **luteinizing hormone** (LH) in males;
4. **Insulins**;
5. **Corticotrophins**; and other substances with similar chemical structure or similar biologic effect(s).

### S3 β-2 agonists
All β-2 agonists including their D- and L-isomers are prohibited.

Therefore, formoterol, salbutamol, salmeterol, and terbutaline when administered by inhalation also require a Therapeutic Use Exemption in accordance with the relevant section of the International Standard for Therapeutic Use Exemptions (WADA TUE).

Despite the granting of a Therapeutic Use Exemption, the presence of salbutamol in urine in excess of 1000 ng/mL will be considered as an *Adverse Analytical Finding* unless the *Athlete* proves, through a controlled pharmacokinetic study, that the abnormal result was the consequence of the use of a therapeutic dose of inhaled salbutamol.

### S4. Hormone antagonists and modulators
The following classes are prohibited:

1. **Aromatase inhibitors** including, but not limited to: **anastrozole, letrozole, aminoglutethimide, exemestane, formestane, testolactone.**
2. **Selective estrogen receptor modulators (SERMs)** including, but not limited to: **raloxifene, tamoxifen, toremifene.**
3. **Other anti-estrogenic substances** including, but not limited to: **clomiphene, cyclofenil, fulvestrant.**
4. **Agents modifying myostatin function(s)** including, but not limited to: **myostatin inhibitors.**

### S5. Diuretics and other masking agents
Masking agents are prohibited. They include:

**Diuretics, probenecid, plasma expanders (**eg, intravenous administration of **albumin, dextran, hydroxyethyl starch**, and **mannitol)** and other substances with similar biologic effect(s).

Diuretics include:

**Acetazolamide, amiloride, bumetanide, canrenone, chlorthalidone, etacrynic acid, furosemide, indapamide, metolazone, spironolactone, thiazides (**eg, **bendroflumethiazide, chlorothiazide, hydrochlorothiazide), triamterene**, and other substances with a similar chemical structure or similar biologic effect(s) (except drosperinone and topical dorzolamide and brinzolamide, which are not prohibited).

### Prohibited Methods

### M1. Enhancement of oxygen transfer
The following are prohibited:

1. Blood doping, including the use of autologous, homologous, or heterologous blood or red blood cell products of any origin.
2. Artificially enhancing the uptake, transport or delivery of oxygen, including but not limited to perfluorochemicals, efaproxiral (RSR13), and modified hemoglobin products (eg, hemoglobin-based blood substitutes, microencapsulated hemoglobin products).

### M2. Chemical and physical manipulation

1. *Tampering,* or attempting to tamper, to alter the integrity and validity of *Samples* collected during *Doping Controls* is prohibited. These include but are not limited to catheterization, urine substitution, and/or alteration.
2. Intravenous infusions are prohibited except in the management of surgical procedures, medical emergencies, or clinical investigations.

### M3. Gene doping

The transfer of cells or genetic elements or the use of cells, genetic elements, or pharmacologic agents to modulating expression of endogenous genes having the capacity to enhance athletic performance, is prohibited.

Peroxisome proliferator activated receptor $\delta$ (PPAR$\delta$) agonists (eg, GW 1516) and PPAR$\delta$-AMP-activated protein kinase (AMPK) axis agonists (eg, AICAR) are prohibited.

## SUBSTANCES AND METHODS PROHIBITED *IN-COMPETITION*

In addition to the categories S1 to S5 and M1 to M3 defined above, the following categories are prohibited in competition:

### Prohibited Substances

### S6. Stimulants

All stimulants (including both their D- and L-optical isomers where relevant) are prohibited, except imidazole derivatives for topical use and those stimulants included in the 2009 Monitoring Program[e].

Stimulants include:

a: Non Specified Stimulants:

Adrafinil; amfepramone; amiphenazole; amphetamine; amphetaminil; benzphetamine; benzylpiperazine; bromantan; clobenzorex; cocaine; cropropamide; crotetamide; dimethylamphetamine; etilamphetamine; famprofazone; fencamine; fenetylline; fenfluramine; fenproporex; furfenorex; mefenorex; mephentermine; mesocarb; methamphetamine(D-); methylenedioxyamphetamine; methylenedioxymethamphetamine; p-methylamphetamine; modafinil; norfenfluramine; phendimetrazine; phenmetrazine; phentermine; 4-phenylpiracetam (carphedon); prolintane.

A stimulant not expressly listed in this section is a Specified Substance.

b: Specified Stimulants (examples):

Adrenaline;[f] cathine;[g] ephedrine;[h] etamivan; etilefrine; fenbutrazate; fencamfamin; heptaminol; isometheptene; levmetamphetamine; meclofenoxate; methylephedrine;[6] methylphenidate; nikethamide; norfenefrine; octopamine;

---

[e] The following substances included in the 2009 Monitoring Program are not considered as *Prohibited Substances*: bupropion, caffeine, phenylephrine, phenylpropanolamine, pipradol, pseudoephedrine, synephrine.

[f] Adrenaline associated with local anesthetic agents or by local administration (eg, nasal, ophthalmologic) is not prohibited.

[g] Cathine is prohibited when its concentration in urine is greater than 5 µg/mL.

[h] Each of ephedrine and methylephedrine is prohibited when its concentration in urine is greater than 10 µg/mL.

oxilofrine; parahydroxyamphetamine; pemoline; pentetrazol; phenprometh-amine; propylhexedrine; selegiline; sibutramine; strychnine; tuaminoheptane and other substances with a similar chemical structure or similar biologic effect(s).

### S7. Narcotics
The following narcotics are prohibited:

**Buprenorphine, dextromoramide, diamorphine (heroin), fentanyl and its derivatives, hydromorphone, methadone, morphine, oxycodone, oxymorphone, pentazocine, pethidine.**

### S8. Cannabinoids
Cannabinoids (eg, hashish, marijuana) are prohibited.

### S9. Glucocorticosteroids
All glucocorticosteroids are prohibited when administered by oral, intravenous, intramuscular, or rectal routes.

In accordance with the International Standard for Therapeutic Use Exemptions, a declaration of use must be completed by the *Athlete* for glucocorticosteroids administered by intra-articular, periarticular, peritendinous, epidural, intradermal, and inhalation routes, except as noted below.

Topical preparations when used for auricular, buccal, dermatologic (including iontophoresis/phonophoresis), gingival, nasal, ophthalmic and perianal disorders are not prohibited and neither require a Therapeutic Use Exemption nor a declaration of use.

### SUBSTANCES PROHIBITED IN PARTICULAR SPORTS
### P1. Alcohol

Alcohol (ethanol) is prohibited *In-competition* only, in the following sports. Detection will be conducted by analysis of breath and/or blood. The doping violation threshold (hematological values) is 0.10 g/L.

- Aeronautic (FAI)
- Archery (FITA, IPC)
- Automobile (FIA)
- Boules (IPC bowls)
- Karate (WKF)
- Modern Pentathlon (UIPM) for disciplines involving shooting
- Motorcycling (FIM)
- Ninepin and Tenpin Bowling (FIQ)
- Powerboating (UIM)

### P2. β-Blockers

Unless otherwise specified, b-blockers are prohibited *In-competition* only, in the following sports.

- Aeronautic (FAI)
- Archery (FITA, IPC) (also prohibited *Out-of-competition*)
- Automobile (FIA)
- Billiards and Snooker (WCBS)
- Bobsleigh (FIBT)
- Boules (CMSB, IPC bowls)
- Bridge (FMB)

- Curling (WCF)
- Golf (IGF)
- Gymnastics (FIG)
- Motorcycling (FIM)
- Modern Pentathlon (UIPM) for disciplines involving shooting
- Ninepin and Tenpin Bowling (FIQ)
- Powerboating (UIM)
- Sailing (ISAF) for match race helms only
- Shooting (ISSF, IPC) (also prohibited *Out-of-competition*)
- Skiing/Snowboarding (FIS) in ski jumping, freestyle aerials/halfpipe and snowboard halfpipe/big air
- Wrestling (FILA)

β-Blockers include, but are not limited to, the following:

**Acebutolol, alprenolol, atenolol, betaxolol, bisoprolol, bunolol, carteolol, carvedilol, celiprolol, esmolol, labetalol, levobunolol, metipranolol, metoprolol, nadolol, oxprenolol, pindolol, propranolol, sotalol, timolol.**

## DRUGS POTENTIALLY ABUSED IN BOXING

It is beyond the scope of this article to specifically address the various drugs that potentially may be abused in boxing. The reasons specific drugs may be used as doping agents are multiple and include, but are not limited to increasing strength and power, increasing lean body mass, decreasing body fat, increasing aggressiveness, improving recovery time, making weight, masking pain, enhancing reaction time, increasing eye-hand coordination, masking fatigue, masking other drugs, and increasing endurance.

## THERAPEUTIC USE EXEMPTIONS

A critical component of anti-doping is the concept of therapeutic use exemptions (TUE). Athletes, like all others, may have illnesses or conditions that may require them to take particular medications.[8] If the medication an athlete is required to take to treat an illness or condition happens to fall under the Prohibited List, a TUE may give that athlete the authorization to take the needed medicine provided that certain rigorous criteria are fulfilled. The TUE protocol is quite precise and harmonized to assure that the process is not abused.

The underlying principles and criteria for granting an athlete a therapeutic use exemption are:

- The athlete would experience significant health problems without taking the prohibited substance or using the prohibited method;
- The therapeutic use of the substance would not produce significant enhancement of performance; and
- There is no reasonable therapeutic alternative to the use of the otherwise prohibited substance or method.

## IN-COMPETITION VERSUS OUT-OF-COMPETITION TESTING (AIBA)

In-competition testing refers to testing when a boxer is selected for testing in connection with a specific competition such as world championships, national tournament, or Olympic Games. For the Amateur International Boxing Association (AIBA), the recognized In-competition testing period begins at midnight the day of the initial draw until midnight the day following the end of the contest.[10]

Out-of-competition testing is any doping control which is—logically—not organized during the recognized period of In-competition testing. Out-of-competition testing can happen anytime and anywhere. It can happen that a boxer is tested by his or her national federation one day and the next day the AIBA turns up once more for another test.

## GOVERNING BODIES

Perhaps more than any other sport there is an array of governing bodies in both amateur and professional boxing, each with its own set of rules and regulations. This situation makes it incumbent on the boxer, whether amateur or professional, to know which anti-doping rules are in effect for any given competition, for example, the World Boxing Council (WBC) and the World Boxing Association (WBA), USA Boxing, or for the various state athletic commissions. This knowledge is imperative, for in doping control the devil is in the details. Such detail pertains not only to the Prohibited List but similarly pertains to the governing body's TUE process and results management protocol, including sanctions.

## SUMMARY

There is nothing in the sport of boxing that makes it immune from doping. Doping is a violation of the public trust and has a corrosive effect on the sport itself. The adverse health effects associated with doping aside, simply stated doping, or taking banned substances for the purpose of enhancing performance, is cheating; it is drug abuse. The possibility that an athlete is doped not only casts doubt on the performance of the individual athlete, it casts doubt on the legitimacy of the sport itself.

Over the past half century, research has enabled remarkable advances in analytical chemistry, permitting anti-doping organizations to identify and sanction athletes who have been doped with an array of pharmaceutical products, the overwhelming majority of which were developed to treat diseases.

As so eloquently stated by the columnist George Will:

*A society's recreation is charged with moral significance. Sport—and a society that takes it seriously—would be debased if it did not strictly forbid things that blur the distinction between the triumph of character and the triumph of chemistry.*[11]

## REFERENCES

1. Lipsyte R. Baseball & drugs. The Nation May 25, 1985. p. 613.
2. Dimeo P. Sports, drugs and society. In: A history of drug use in sport. Beyond good an evil. London: Routledge; 2007. p. 7.
3. Catlin DH, Fitch KD, Ljungqvist A. Medicine and science in the fight against doping in sport. J Intern Med 2008;264:99–114.
4. Thompson T, Vinton L. Victor conte files counter to shane Mosley suit. New York Daily News; Dec 24, 2008.
5. Fainaru-Wada M, Williams M. Game of Shadows. New York: Gotham Books; 2006.
6. WBC looks into Mosley's testimony to grand jury. Canada.com. Agence France Presse; Dec 17, 2008.
7. World Anti-Doping Agency. Available at: www.wada-ama.org.
8. World Anti-Doping Code. World Anti-Doping Agency; 2009.

9. World Anti-Doping Code. Montreal, Quebec: World Anti-Doping Agency; 2009. p. 18–25.

10. AIBA anti-doping 2009. Available at: http://www.aiba.org/default.aspx?pId=167.

11. Wadler GI, Hainline B. Anabolic steroids. In: Drugs and the athlete. Philadelphia: FA Davis; 1989. p. 67.

# Infectious Disease and Boxing

Osric S. King, MD[a,b,*]

KEYWORDS

- Boxing illnesses • Boxing respiratory diseases
- Boxing airborne infections • Boxing dermatologic infections

There are no unique boxing diseases but certain factors contributing to the spread of illnesses apply strongly to the boxer, coach, and the training facility. Like many athletes, boxers spend long hours preparing alone as well as with other boxers and coaches. The very nature of the exercise, surrounding environment, and final competition can increase the likelihood of infection through airborne, contact, and blood-borne routes of transmission. In addition, boxing is one of the unique sports in which the audience can potentially become contaminated and exposed to certain diseases. Fortunately, there have been no documented disease outbreaks associated with the sport. Also, the gross underreporting of boxing illnesses in the literature makes discussions of these situations more speculative than evidence-based. This article includes evidence from other sports such as running, wrestling, and martial arts to help elucidate the pathophysiologic elements that could be identified in boxers.

## IMMUNE SYSTEM PHYSIOLOGY

Often, before an important fight a boxer is isolated from his usual environment in an attempt to enhance his focus by minimizing distractions. The additional benefit of the seclusion is that it minimizes exposure to potential infectious agents that could jeopardize his or her health before an important fight. Vigorous physical exertion produces alterations in the body's ability to fight infection.[1] The circulatory system stimulates the changes in the immune system on several levels affecting the skin cells, upper respiratory tract mucosa, lung, peritoneal cavity, and muscles. Exercise-induced stress affects the natural killer cells, neutrophils, and macrophages. Changes occur by influencing stress hormones, cytokine concentration, body temperature, blood flow, and hydration. The result is immune dysfunction lasting 3 to 72 hours. This dysfunction provides organisms a window of opportunity to increase the risk of subclinical and clinical infection.[1,2] The overall effect appears to be modified by the degree of stress.[3] There is an increased risk associated with heavy training, whereas moderate training has been associated with a reduction in upper respiratory tract

[a] Hospital for Special Surgery, 535 East 70th Street New York, NY 10021, USA
[b] New York State Athletic Commission
* Corresponding author. Hospital for Special Surgery, 535 East 70th Street, New York, NY 10021.
*E-mail address:* kingo@hss.edu

Clin Sports Med 28 (2009) 545–560
doi:10.1016/j.csm.2009.06.002
0278-5919/09/$ – see front matter © 2009 Published by Elsevier Inc.

sportsmed.theclinics.com

infection (URTI) incidence. The risk of infection can also be amplified by the additional factors related to severe mental stress, sleep deprivation, and weight loss when a fighter has to make the necessary weight for an event.[4]

Hydration is a critical element for the body's immune system and there is evidence to suggest that dehydration can predispose an individual to developing a fever.[5] In addition to being in optimal physical and mental condition, a boxer must make the weight stipulated by his division for the event. Because fat and muscle cannot be reduced quickly, dehydration becomes the main tool for losing a few pounds. The process can occur over a few months, weeks, days and, unfortunately, hours. Steam baths, plastic suits, laxatives, vomiting, and expectoration are used individually or in combination to achieve the desired weight loss. This activity can produce a potentially dangerous situation in regard to the boxer's susceptibility to infection. The mucosal layer of the oral pharynx is one of the first lines of protection from an invading organism. Exposure from the acidic contents of the stomach that occurs during induced vomiting directly compromises this barrier. In addition, diminishing the volume of saliva will also deplete the quantity of immunoglobulin A available to protect the oral and respiratory tract. Further volume depletion by the other methods can increase the heart rate and induce stress during a time when the boxer is relatively inactive. This stress can influence the body's ability to fight infection.

Diet and nutrition can play a role in counteracting some of the detrimental effects of exercise on the immune system. Water is the life blood of an active boxer during training and competition. Water is essential for providing the necessary hydration during exercise. Unfortunately, it contains none of the calories, proteins, or electrolytes necessary to enhance immune system function. Ingestion of carbohydrate beverages during intense and prolonged exercise seems effective in mitigating exercise-induced immune suppression.[6] In addition, protein intake can increase insulin levels, optimize glycogen resynthesis, and enhance protein production necessary to fight infection.[7] The use of some supplements such as quercetin also have the potential to lessen the magnitude of exercise-induced perturbations in immune function and reduce the risk of URTIs.[8] Quercetin is found in onions, blueberries, curly kale, hot peppers, tea, and broccoli. Not only is quercetin a powerful antioxidant but it seems to also exert antipathogenic activity against a variety of viruses and bacteria. Other supplements such as vitamins E and C have not shown meaningful effects on exercise-induced inflammation, muscle damage, increases in plasma cytokines, and immune perturbations.[9,10]

In total, the physiologic effects of training seem to be more of a benefit then detriment because most conditioned athletes do not appear to experience any infectious diseases at a greater prevalence than the general population.

## ENVIRONMENT

Intense training produces blood, sweat, and tears, which are among the nicer things found in a boxing gym. In studies, biochemical markers for blood, mucous, saliva, sweat, feces, and urine were detected on 36% of the surfaces in a daycare center.[11] It is conceivable that in a gym wherein hygiene and hand washing are not emphasized, most surfaces will be contaminated. Locations such as the ring mat and ropes make contact with every external part of the human anatomy unprotected, or sponged through shirts and shorts soaked with a combination of water, blood, perspiration, urine, and saliva. Objects frequently struck such as speed or heavy bags can provide an effective means for making fungus, bacteria, and viruses airborne. To complicate matters, items such as boxing gloves, head gear, and protective gonad cups are infrequently sanitized with disinfectant and can act as infectious reservoirs. Fortunately, most boxers routinely shower after their workout, which theoretically can diminish the bacterial or viral load present on the epidermis especially if certain soaps are used.[12]

## AIRBORNE INFECTIONS

Similar to other individuals, the most likely illness a boxer will face is an URTI. Most of theses infections are from viruses but it is important to recognize bacterial infections and their potential complications. Also, supportive care for a viral infection should be selected carefully so as to avoid potentially dangerous reactions when symptom control medications are used during exercise activities.

The second most common illness seen in a United States physician's office is the common cold.[13] The initial symptoms consist of sore throat, malaise, and low-grade fever. These symptoms may resolve in a few days and are followed by rhinorrhea, cough, and nasal congestion. The symptoms usually peak around day three or four and usually resolve by day seven.[14] Rhinovirus is the most common source but the common cold can be caused by one of several viruses including coronavirus, respiratory syncytial virus, influenza virus, parainfluenza virus, and adenovirus. There are no effective antivirals to cure the common cold and few effective measures to prevent it. Antibiotics are inappropriately prescribed to improve cure rate and symptom persistence, and prevent secondary bacterial complications. Systematic reviews have shown that antibiotics are ineffective in controlling symptoms and have no role in the treatment of the common cold.[15,16] Furthermore, antibiotics increase the risk of gastrointestinal effects, allergic reactions, and resistance of bacteria to antibiotics. Treatment of a cold should focus on controlling the symptoms. Nontraditional complementary and alternative therapies used for the common cold include *Echinacea*, vitamin C, zinc, and humidified air and fluid intake.[17] Two well-conducted studies and a Cochrane review showed no benefit from using *Echinacea* to treat or prevent the common cold.[18–20] There is no evidence that vitamin C decreases symptom severity or duration when initiated after the onset of cold symptoms. However, when used prophylactically, an exercise group taking vitamin C had a 50% relative reduction in the risk of developing a cold. Studies with zinc show inconsistent viral growth inhibition and reduction of cold symptoms duration.[21] The use of humidified air and fluid intake are considered benign and possibly beneficial for the relief of common cold symptoms.[16] A Cochrane review showed some evidence that dextromethorphan provided a modest clinical benefit controlling coughs. Overall, however, there is a lack of evidence to determine the effectiveness of any over-the-counter product at reducing the frequency or severity of cough in children or adults.[22] The American College of Chest Physicians guidelines do not recommend centrally acting cough suppressants (codeine or dextromethorphan) for cough secondary to URTI.[23] For nasal congestion and rhinorrhea symptoms, antihistamines remain a popular therapy and the older first-generation products have shown positive results for certain end points. However, a Cochrane review concluded that antihistamines do not alleviate cold-related sneezing or nasal symptoms to a clinically significant degree, and do not affect subjective improvement in children or adults.[24] Studies appear to support the short-term use of intranasal and oral decongestants as well as the use of topical ipratropium (Atrovent) for rhinorrhea.[16] Extreme symptoms may warrant the use of some antihistamines, decongestants, dextromethorphan and, most importantly, rest. Antihistamines, dextromethorphan, and decongestants, even without exertion, can cause cardiac arrhythmias, blurred vision, hypertension, seizures, respiratory depression, irritability, confusion and irritability, and sedation.[16] In a boxer, the use of these medications combined with rigorous training, let alone a fight, could be potentially fatal. There are also studies relating a risk of stroke to the over-the-counter cough and cold drugs. The mechanism seems related to hypertension or vasospasm or angiitis.[25] Overall, the gain in taking cold symptom medication to train or perform more comfortably does not outweigh the potential risk from the side effects.

### Acute Sinusitis

Acute sinusitis is defined as the inflammation of the mucosal lining of the paranasal sinuses lasting less than 4 weeks. Viral URTI is often the trigger for bacterial sinusitis,[26] with about 0.5% of common colds becoming complicated by the development of acute sinusitis.[27] Viral infection is the most common cause of acute sinusitis, and usually resolves in 7 to 10 days. Acute bacterial sinusitis is also self-limiting, with 75% of cases resolving without treatment within 1 month.[28] The usual pathogens are *Streptococcus pneumoniae* and *Haemophilus influenzae* with occasional infection with *Moraxella catarrhalis*. The diagnosis is most commonly based on clinical history and physical findings. Laboratory tests can assist in chronic or complicated cases but imaging studies may not be useful because asymptomatic sinusitis is often reported on a boxer's magnetic resonance imaging (MRI) or computed tomography (CT) scans. The symptoms consist of nasal congestion, purulent nasal discharge, maxillary tooth discomfort, headaches, fever, and facial pain or pressure that is worse when leaning forward. Treatment is often sought when training is complicated by the inability to breathe through the nose. This situation helps to distinguish traumatic headache from sinus headache. Left untreated, some bacterial sinusitis may not spontaneously resolve and can have severe complications including intracranial and orbital infections. Superimposed facial trauma could potentially predispose or advance the disease. The use of cephalosporins and macrolides seem to be as effective as, and have fewer adverse effects than amoxicillin or amoxicillin-clavulanate. Intranasal corticosteroid sprays and decongestants may be effective in reducing symptoms. There do not appear to be any studies supporting the effectiveness of decongestants, antihistamines, saline nasal washes, and steam inhalation in reducing the duration of the illnesses.[29] However, the latter two treatments offer the most benefit and the least risk of adverse effects.

### Pharyngitis

When eating or swallowing food is painful, most boxers will seek medical attention. Although most sore throats have an infectious origin, fewer than 20% have a clear indication for antibiotic therapy. Bacterial pathogens include group C and group G *Streptococcus*, mixed anaerobes, *Corynebacterium diphtheria*, and several chlamydial species. The major common pathogen warranting treatment is Group A b-hemolytic streptococcus (GABHS), which accounts for 5% to 15% of cases and, infrequently, can be responsible for rheumatic fever, acute glomerulonephritis, and peritonsillar abscess.[30] Pharyngeal swelling, tonsillar exudates, fever, and tender anterior cervical lymph nodes and a scarlet rash suggest GABHS infection. Laboratory analysis clarifies the decision to treat with antibiotics. Throat cultures remain the gold standard for confirming the diagnosis, with sensitivity approaching 97% and specificity ranging from 95% to 99%.[31] Rapid antigen detection tests are almost as sensitive as throat cultures. These tests are readily available and easy to perform, with results available within minutes.[32] When individuals fail to improve with antibiotic treatment, other origins of their symptoms may include mononucleosis and possibly gastroesophageal reflux. In boxers who are sexually active and present with fever, sore throat, dysuria, and characteristic greenish exudates, gonococcal pharyngitis should be considered.[33] A rash following the administration of antibiotics can indicate a drug allergy or possible viral infection with mononucleosis. In addition to high fever, pharyngitis, and lymphadenopathy, the boxer with mononucleosis may classically present with extreme fatigue (especially after the acute symptoms have resolved). Laboratory analysis is important in confirming the disease and may show atypical lymphocytes, elevated mononucleosis titers, and elevated liver function tests. Testing during mild symptoms or early in the episode may yield a false positive. A major risk for boxers is the possibility of splenomegaly and subsequent splenic rupture with activity. The incidence of splenic rupture is 1 to 2 cases per 1000,[34] and occurs spontaneously in half of the cases between the fourth and 21st days of symptomatic illness.[35] The major concern is that direct thoracic and abdominal blows are expected in boxing and could be fatal in the presence of splenomegaly. Ultrasound evaluation of the spleen size is of some value but 7% of athletes' baseline spleen size meets the current criteria for splenomegaly.[36] Another concern for mononucleosis is its long incubation period and potential for asymptomatic spread. Contamination occurs through contact with saliva. This contact may occur directly through the sharing of water bottles or possibly indirectly because saliva may be present on gloves, ropes, or other surfaces.

### Community-Acquired Pneumonia

The term community-acquired pneumonia (CAP) is used when the patient has not been hospitalized or in a long-term facility for at least 14 days before the onset of symptoms. The symptoms include cough, fever, chills, fatigue, dyspnea, rigors, and pleuritic chest pain. The expected musculoskeletal discomfort from training could make the early detection of pneumonia difficult in a boxer. Origins such as *Legionella* may also produce gastrointestinal symptoms. Typical pneumonia is caused by *Streptococcus pneumoniae* and is found in very young or older patients. Atypical pneumonias are found most often in young adults and are usually caused by influenza virus, *Mycoplasma*, *Legionella*, *Chlamydia*, and adenovirus.[37] Chest radiography is the gold standard in diagnosing pneumonia but may show as falsely negative early in the disease. The validity of common laboratory tests such as leukocyte count, sputum stain, and blood cultures have been questioned after low positive culture rates were found.[38] Antibiotics that provide coverage against the most common organisms known to cause CAP should be used for treatment.

### Bronchitis

Acute bronchitis is inflammation of the bronchial mucus membranes. Acute bronchitis should be suspected when a boxer presents coughing with or without sputum lasting up to 3 weeks with evidence of concurrent upper airway infection. The most common cause is viral infections. Less than 10% have bacterial origin. The most common viruses are influenza A and B, adenovirus, rhinovirus, parainfluenza virus, coronavirus, and respiratory syncytial virus. The bacteria found in acute bronchitis are *Bordetella pertussis*, *Mycoplasma pneumoniae* and *Chlamydia pneumoniae*.[39] Despite improvements in testing and technology, diagnosis of bronchitis is mostly clinical because no routinely performed procedures diagnose acute bronchitis. Chest radiography should be reserved for use in patients whose physical examination suggest pneumonia or heart failure, and in patients who would be at high risk if the diagnosis were delayed.[40] The recommended therapy is symptomatic care if the clinical diagnosis of acute bronchitis is established. Treatment should focus on preventing or controlling the cough (antitussive therapy) or on making the cough more effective (protussive therapy). Terbutaline, amiloride, and hypertonic saline aerosols have proved successful in protussive treatment of coughs from various causes. Studies with guaifenesin were inconclusive because the dose evaluated was less than what is usually prescribed.[41]

Antitussive selection is based on the cause of the cough. An antihistamine would be used to treat cough associated with allergic rhinitis, a decongestant or an antihistamine would be selected for cough associated with postnasal drainage, and a bronchodilator would be appropriate for cough associated with asthma- and nonasthma-related conditions.[42] Nonspecific antitussives such as hydrocodone, dextromethorphan, and codeine simply suppress cough and their side effects should be considered when a boxer is training.

### Pericarditis

In a boxer it is crucial to distinguish between cardiac chest pain and training-related musculoskeletal soreness. Pericarditis is the inflammation of the pericardium, the sac surrounding the heart. Pericarditis is most often secondary to a viral infection but it may also be caused by other diseases, drugs, invasive cardiothoracic procedures, and chest trauma.[43] Symptoms may be mild with no significant discomfort or they might present with sudden onset of severe substernal chest pain. Viral origins include coxsackievirus A and B, hepatitis viruses, human immunodeficiency virus (HIV), influenza, measles, mumps, and *Varicella*. Bacterial causes include gram-positive and gram-negative organisms and, rarely, *Mycobacterium tuberculosis*. Fungal origins are seen in immunocompromised patients: *Blastomyces dermatidis*, *Candida*, and *Histoplasma capsulatum*. A boxer may present with a history of fever, malaise, and myalgias. The cardinal features of acute pericarditis are chest pain, which is left-sided and may radiate to the trapezius, neck, arms, or jaws. With this pain distribution in mind, it is understandable that the symptoms are easily misinterpreted; this is especially true after extensive training. The detection of pericardial friction rub on auscultation has a high specificity but a low sensitivity that varies with the frequency of auscultation.[44] The electrocardiogram is abnormal in 90% of pericarditis cases.[45] Laboratory analysis may show evidence of inflammation with elevated C-reactive protein, erythrocyte sedimentation rate and leukocyte count. Markers of myocardial injury such as the MB isoenzyme of creatine kinase and cardiac troponins are also elevated. Echocardiography may be normal, CT and MRI are useful if the initial workup for pericarditis is inconclusive.[46] The goal of treatment is to relieve pain and prevent complications such as recurrence, tamponade and chronic restrictive pericarditis. Whether to manage the patient as an outpatient or inpatient will depend on the level of complications and severity.

### Myocarditis

Another source of cardiac chest pain in a boxer is myocarditis, which is the inflammation of the cardiac muscle. Myocarditis is most commonly caused by viruses such as coxsackievirus B, adenovirus, hepatitis C virus, cytomegalovirus, echovirus, influenza virus, and Epstein-Barr virus. The boxer may be asymptomatic, giving a history of a preceding URTI, or he might present with symptoms of chest pain or heart failure. The physical examination may reveal a muffled first heart sound along with a third heart sound and a murmur of mitral regurgitation. Lower extremity edema along with pulmonary crackles from fluid overload may indicate the severity of the condition. Routine blood tests are generally normal but creatine kinase-MB and troponin I may be elevated. Electrocardiographic findings are transient and may show nonspecific ST-T wave abnormalities. Chest radiographs may show pulmonary congestion and cardiomegaly. Echocardiograms are useful and may reveal global decreased ventricle dysfunction. Treatment is generally supportive for viral causes with the emphasis on treating heart failure and potential arrhythmias in serious cases.[47] Following the acute illness, myocarditis as well as pericarditis can cause 11% of sudden and unexpected cardiac death during or after physical exercise.[48] Surprisingly, some individuals are asymptomatic.[49] Because of this danger, Bethesda Conference recommends that athletes who have probable or definitive evidence of myocarditis should be withdrawn from all competitive sports and undergo a prudent convalescent period of about 6 months.

## CONTACT INFECTIONS

Skin infections are often the result of a break in the integrity of the skin. The organism can be fungi, virus, or bacteria. Most boxers will experience facial lacerations during the course of their career. What contaminates the wound depends on two factors: the organism colonizing the skin or glove before impact and what was used to control the bleeding that followed. Ideally, sterile gauze applied by an experienced "cut man" using a swab will be applied to the lesion. It is likely that the "corner towel" previously used to absorb the boxer's perspiration and possibly wipe water from the mat is implemented to achieve hemostasis. With this in mind, there is enormous potential for infections.

### Fungus

In boxing, the skin's mechanisms of protection fails because of repeated trauma, irritation, and maceration during the course of training. In addition, skin occlusion with nonporous materials, seen with some protective head and gonad gear, interfere with the skin's barrier function. This interference occurs by increasing local temperature and hydration.[50] In wrestlers, fungal infections, termed tinea corporis gladitorum, can be seen in up to 75% of participants. The transmission is primarily through skin-to-skin contact. Lesions are typically found on the head, neck, and arms.[51] Although there is different, and relatively less, contact made in boxing compared with wrestling, the potential for contamination exists. *Microsporum*, *Trichophyton*, and *Epidermophyton* species are the most common fungal pathogens in skin infections. These pathogens are categorized as dermatophytes or tinea because they are fungi that require keratin (found in skin, hair, and nails) for growth. Superficial skin infections are caused less frequently by nondermatophyte fungi such as *Malassezia furfur* in tinea/pityriasis versicolor, and *Candida* species. Transmission can occur by direct contact or from exposure to desquamated cells. Inoculation occurs through breaks in the skin. Germination occurs following the invasion of the superficial skin layers. The physical examination typically reveals an inflammatory response characterized by a greater degree of redness and scaling at the edge of the lesion or occasionally by blister formation. Potassium hydroxide (KOH) microscopy aids in visualizing hyphae and confirming the diagnosis of dermatophyte infection. Other diagnostic modalities include Wood's lamp examination, fungal culture, and skin or nail biopsy.[52] Topical treatment is usually adequate for most tinea except tinea capitis, tinea barbae, tinea unguium and, rarely, tinea corporis.

### Virus

Sexual activity, skin-to-skin contact, and the contaminated surfaces of a gym are high-risk routes of viral infection. Molluscum contagiosum (MC), human papillomavirus (HPV), and herpes are the most likely viruses to infect the skin of a boxer.

MC infections occur frequently among children and also affect sexually active adults.[53] MC may also serve as a cutaneous marker of severe immunodeficiency and sometimes is the first indication of HIV infection.[54] MC is a double-stranded DNA virus in the Poxviridae family. MC is spread through fomite or skin-to-skin contact, and abrasions in the epidermis are thought to facilitate transmission.[55] The typical appearance is an asymptomatic, firm, smooth, round papule with central umbilication, typically found on the extremities, trunk, and face. In sexually transmitted cases they can be found on the lower abdomen and in the genital region. Spontaneous resolution of the lesions occurs but eradication is possible through mechanical (curettage, laser, cryotherapy), chemical (trichloroacetic acid, tretinoin), or immunologic (imiquimod) means.

Human papillomavirus causes warts that can occur almost anywhere on the body. After initial infection by direct contact from skin or a contaminated surface, warts are frequently spread by autoinoculation from scratching, shaving, or skin trauma. The appearance may vary from an irregularly surfaced domed lesion (common warts) to a filiform projection seen on the face, to flat plantar warts on the plantar surface of feet. Plantar warts tend to be painful because they become callused and grow into the foot instead of rising above the surface. Treatment options for warts include mechanical destruction and adjustment of the patient's immune system through medications.

Skin infection with herpes simplex virus (HSV) poses a huge risk to boxers. HSV affects more than one-third of the world's population and is responsible for a wide array of symptoms, and may occasionally lead to death. There are two separate types, labeled HSV-1 and HSV-2. Each type has affinities for different body sites. HSV-1 causes 90% of oral lesions and HSV-2 causes 90% of genital lesions. Both viruses enter the host through abraded skin or intact mucous membranes. Epithelial cells are the initial targets. Once infected these cells die, releasing clear fluid intradermally to form vesicles. Retrograde transport through adjacent neural tissue to sensory ganglia leads to lifelong latent infection.[56] The initial infection is usually due to skin-to-skin contact. Transmission can potentially occur from inanimate objects, as in the case of an English boxer whose glove, contaminated with smallpox, was reported to infect his Norwegian opponent in 1948.[57] HSV has been reported to survive on plastic spa surfaces at temperatures around 100°F (38°C) for up to 4.5 minutes.[58] To complicate matters further, asymptomatic shedding of viral particles happens frequently, making infection identification and prevention based on visualizing lesions extremely ineffective. Reactivation of the virus causes recurrent symptoms and is triggered by local or systemic stimuli such as ultraviolet light (UV), trauma, fever, and immunodeficiency. During training, a boxer may be exposed to all of these factors individually or in combination. Latent HSV-1 may reactivate in boxers during exposure to UV light from the sun that may occur during running or "road work."[59] Trauma from punches to the face, with and without head gear, during sparring sessions could also contribute to developing HSV-1 lesions. Physical and mental stress can induce immune suppression and has been shown to increase HSV-associated pathogenicity. Once HSV is located in a boxer's skin, the incubation period ranges from a few days to several weeks. First a prodrome characterized by burning, stinging, itching, or pain in the area, eventually develops into a skin lesion. Very early lesions have a nonspecific clinical appearance, usually as well-defined erythematous papules. As the individual lesions resolve, a crust develops on top. Systemic symptoms are not unusual, especially in cases of primary HSV infection. Athletes may complain of fever, sore throat, malaise, myalgias, arthralgias, and swollen lymph nodes. The recurrent symptoms around the face are usually self-limiting without treatment. The potential for eye and central nervous system involvement is the greatest risk for boxers. Involvement of the eye (including conjunctivitis, blepharitis, and keratitis) has been well documented in wrestlers.[60] There is also a documented case of a rugby player developing HSV-related meningitis and sacral ganglionitis with perineal and lower extremity paresthesias.[61] Acyclovir, famciclovir, and valacyclovir are the main antivirals used for treating

HSV infections. There are financial and convenience factors involved in deciding which medication to use. Overall, treatment is valuable because it lessens the pain, degree of viral shedding, constitutional symptoms, and lesion healing time.

### Bacterial

Second to HIV, there is arguably no infectious organism that has received as much recent publicity as methicillin-resistant *Staphylococcus aureus* (MRSA). MRSA infections have been a complication in hospital settings for over 40 years.[62] Hospitalization with some degree of immunosuppression and antibiotic use were previously key predisposing factors. In the past few years its presence outside health care centers in immunocompetent individuals with no history of antibiotic use has made MRSA a media favorite. The presence of MRSA in training facilities and in some popular athletes has forced the entire sports community to look closely at current hygienic practices. High school, collegiate, and professional sports have published case reports. Although contact sports such as football, wrestling, and rugby have the most documented cases, infections in athletes participating in basketball, fencing, and weightlifting have also been reported.[63] At the time of writing there were no cases of MRSA in a boxer and only one incidence of a mixed martial arts (MMA) fighter competing with an MRSA infection, which was diagnosed after the event. Thinking he was suffering the effects of rapid weight loss, the athlete ignored signs of fever and vomiting before the fight.[64] Supersaturation of the stratum corneum (the first outer layer of skin) by sweating combined with abrasions and cuts allow the entrance of the microorganism through the epidermis. There is also some link to environmental surfaces, whirlpools, taping gel, and towels.[65,66] There have been no case reports of MRSA in boxing, possibly reflecting underreporting because the predisposing factors exist in abundance. The lesions can present in the form of impetigo, folliculitis, or furunculosis. There are also some reports of periorbital cellulitis in the nonathletic population. Impetigo lesions are characterized by well-defined erythematous papules and plaques with honey-colored crust, with or without pustules. These lesions can also present with discrete clear fluid-filled vesicles that coalesce into larger bullae. The infection can occur with skin-to-skin contact and can be spread further by scratching. Culture confirms the diagnosis. Impetigo can be treated with warm soaks and topical antibiotics but extensive disease necessitates oral antibiotics. Folliculitis is hair follicles that become inflamed by physical injury, chemical irritation, or infection. The hair shaft is frequently be seen in the center of the pustule. Furuncles and carbuncles can occur as follicular infections or impetigo progress deeper. Such a lesion is commonly known as an abscess or boil, and consists of a tender, erythematous, firm, or fluctuant mass of walled-off purulent material. Constitutional symptoms including fever and malaise are common. Treatment often consists of incision and drainage accompanied by oral or, in severe cases, parenteral antibiotics. For most of the bacterial skin lesions, return to sporting activity is after 48 to 72 hours of systemic antibiotics and no new or active draining lesions may be evident at the time of activity.[67]

## BLOODBORNE INFECTION

HIV, hepatitis B virus (HBV), and hepatitis C virus (HCV) are the most common bloodborne pathogens. Boxers are at high risk of spreading or contracting an infection because bleeding occurs frequently during competition. The mechanism of transmission is similar to the general population, and can include using a contaminated needle as well as direct contact from an infected boxer to the opponent's damaged skin or a mucous membrane. In boxing there are several precautions in place to limit the spread of these diseases. The professional boxing commissions in most US states require mandatory periodic testing for these diseases before allowing professional boxers to compete. The amateur boxing supervising authority (USA Boxing) has taken measures to limit excessive bleeding during competition but does not test for infections.

### Human Immunodeficiency Virus

HIV replicates in human cells expressing the T4 (CD4) antigen and causes suppression of the immune system. The individual with HIV has weakened defenses against invading organisms and is susceptible to opportunistic infections which, left untreated, ultimately lead to death. HIV created a huge dilemma for boxing and the other sports in which bleeding can occur. After concerned physicians advocated safer protocols, mandatory testing was initiated early followed by recommendations to stop a bout until bleeding was controlled.[68,69] Safety measures such as universal precautions and mandatory testing were incorporated quickly by most boxing commissions. In boxing, guidelines for excessive bleeding were easy to implement because controlling bleeding is always an important objective for strategic and psychological reasons. Excessive blood cannot only impair vision but distract a boxer if he is constantly trying to wipe it away. Some boxers will also display diminished skills at the sight of their own blood. Overall, the two preventative strategies of testing and bleeding control seem effective in minimizing the incidence of boxing-related transmission of HIV. There is no evidence that HIV can be transmitted through saliva, sweat, or tears,[68] so there is no danger associated with normal body contact such as touching and sharing sports equipment or towels. Also, contaminated surfaces such as ring mats, toilet seats, and hot tubs do not pose risks. According to the US Centers for Disease Control and Prevention (CDC), the risk of transmission of HIV during sports is small and there are no documented cases of HIV contamination during sports.[70] Evidence exists suggesting that the baseline risk of HIV may be higher in competitive athletes. This evidence seems more related to "risky" lifestyle behavior including increased alcohol consumption, inconsistent contraceptive use, and multiple sex partners than the inherent risks of the sport.[71] Intramuscular injection of anabolic steroids and other performance-enhancing drugs constitutes another HIV risk behavior associated with athletes. The case of a body builder with acquired immune deficiency syndrome (AIDS) suggests that like in the general population, contaminated needles are also a source of HIV infection.[72] There is a report of HIV seroconversion as a result of bleeding during a soccer match in Italy.[73] After further investigation, transmission through nonsports activity could not be ruled out because the man involved also worked in a drug dependency rehabilitation program. There are also some case reports of HIV transmission during bloody street fights.[74,75] These events should not be compared with boxing, because they lack the rules and regulations that minimize the dangers and limit morbidity and mortality. Evidence of HIV infection can be found by testing for the antibodies (enzyme-linked immunosorbent assay [ELISA] and Western blot test). Unfortunately, the tests do not become positive until 3 to 4 weeks (sometimes even months) after infection. Quantifying HIV RNA level (viral load) by polymerase chain reaction (PCR), which is 95% to 98% sensitive for HIV, becomes positive within 11 days of infection.[76] At present the ELISA and Western blot tests are the accepted screening tests for boxing. A possible way to strengthen the current protocols may be by mandating viral load testing and including amateur as well as professional boxers. Justifying a change in tests may not be easy because antibody testing is the accepted standard and seems to be working well. There is no denying that that in amateur bouts the chance of HIV transmission through lacerations is less, but not impossible, with the use of headgear. However, nose bleeds are very common and could increase the risk of transmission. Testing amateur boxers may not be cost effective but it would make the disease-screening process more thorough. There is some opinion that the physical demands of the sport would limit participation by athletes infected with HIV.[77] The opposite may be true, with the exertion from boxing training potentially being beneficial for an individual with HIV.[78] Finally, with the current regimen of medications that are able to minimize the viral loads, a boxer with HIV may be able to compete without any obvious limitations and it may not be detectable with the current screening methods. There is a famous case of a boxer diagnosed with HIV who continues to fight professionally. His case is unusual because his initial test was reported positive but subsequent tests have all been negative. It is uncertain whether he was the victim of a false positive, or for whatever reasons, his virus is presently undetectable. At present most professional boxing commissions are not willing to take a chance and allow him to continue competing in their states.

## Hepatitis B Virus

The most common mode of HBV transmission is via intimate sexual contact. When considering direct contact with blood, it is more likely than HIV to be transmitted during boxing because it is present in higher concentrations in the blood and more stable in the environment outside of the body and laboratory. HBV outbreaks in sports are not uncommon and contact with open wounds of HBV carriers is thought to be the precipitating factor. Five of 10 members of a Japanese high school sumo wrestling club contracted hepatitis during a single year. In 2000 an American football team reported that 11 of 65 athletes were found to have HBV over a 19-month period. Most recently, a study revealed 9 of 70 Turkish Olympic wrestlers to have occult HBV infection. The study suggested that sweat may be another way of transmitting HBV infections. At the time writing, two world championship fights were called off because one of the participants was found to have HBV.[79,80] The presence of certain antigens detected by laboratory analysis can determine past, current, or chronic HBV infections (**Box 1**).[81]

---

**Box 1**
**Determination of past, current, or chronic hepatitis B virus infections by laboratory testing for antigens**

*Hepatitis B surface antigen* (HBsAg): Present in acute or chronic infection

*Hepatitis B surface antibody* (anti-HBS): Marker of immunity acquired through natural HBV infection, vaccination or passive antibody

*Hepatitis B core antibody* (anti-HBc):

   IgM—indicates infection in the previous 6 months

   IgG—indicates prior HBV infection that may have been cleared by the immune system or that may persist; positive HBsAg and anti-HBc

   IgG—indicates persistent chronic HBV infection

*Hepatitis Be antigen* (HBeAg): Marker of infectivity that correlates with high viral replication

*Hepatitis Be antibody* (anti-HBe): Correlates with low viral replication

*HBV DNA*: Correlates with active replication; useful in monitoring treatment responses

A boxer with HBV may be asymptomatic or present with myalgia, urticaria, joint pain, nausea, anorexia, low-grade fever, or abdominal pain. Patients may be treated with immune modulators such as interferon or antivirals. No information is available at this time regarding whether boxers treated for HBV can safely return to competition. Many American-born children are vaccinated for HBV, which will help to minimize the prevalence of HBV in the future.

### Hepatitis C Virus

HCV is the most common bloodborne infection, the leading cause of hepatocellular carcinoma, and the principal diagnosis among patients referred for liver transplantation. Acute HCV infection is rarely severe and usually asymptomatic. The virus is transmitted through exposure to infected blood and in the sports world most known transmissions have occurred through shared needles. One observed case involved the injection of anabolic androgenic steroids.[82] Another report involved three amateur soccer players infected with HCV after sharing a syringe to inject vitamin complexes.[83] There was a case in 2000 in which HCV was transmitted during a bloody fight between two family members. At the end of the fight they shared a handkerchief to dry their blood so it is uncertain when the inoculation occurred, during the fight or afterwards. The diagnosis is made by antibody (anti-HCV) testing, which is 99% sensitive and 99% specific. Anti-HCV determines whether a person was exposed but does not detect the presence of active infection. Because some individuals spontaneously clear the infection, the presence of HCV RNA (quantitatively or qualitatively) is used for confirmation. False-negative results for HCV antibody testing may occur in immunosuppressed persons.

### SUMMARY

Boxers are at increased risks for certain infectious diseases because of certain training, environmental, and sociologic parameters. The intensive mental and physical stresses of the sport can alter the ability to fight off disease. The inappropriate use of medications for upper respiratory infections may do more harm than good. The training facility may also influence what fungi, viruses, and bacteria are present to cause infections. Like other sports, dangerous bloodborne diseases are acquired by risky behavior, particularly sexual, and sharing needles to inject performance-enhancing drugs. Precautions are necessary to detect and prevent the spread of illnesses to both participants and observers of boxing. There are treatment options available but the risks and side effects must be weighed against the potential benefits. For some diseases treatment does not guarantee a return to competitive sport.

### REFERENCES

1. Nieman DC. Marathon training and immune function. Sports Med 2007;37(4–5): 412–5.
2. Kruger K, Mooren FC. T cell homing and exercise. Exerc Immunol Rev 2007;13: 37–54.
3. Nieman DC. Exercise and resistance to infection. Can J Physiol Pharmacol 1998; 76(5):573–80.
4. Nieman DC. Special feature for the olympics: effects of exercise on the immune system: exercise effects on systemic immunity. Immunol Cell Biol 2000;78(50): 496–501.
5. Morimoto A, Murahami N, Ono T, et al. Dehydration enhances endotoxin fever by increased production of endogenous pyrogen. Am J Physiol 1986;25(1 Pt 2):R41–7.

6. Walker GJ, Finlay O, Griffiths H, et al. Immunoendocrine response to cycling following injestion of caffeine and carbohydrate. Med Sci Sports Exerc 2007; 39(9):1554–60.
7. Kreider RB, Earnest CP, Lundberg J, et al. Effects of ingesting protein with various forms of carbohydrate following resistance-exercise on substrate availability and markers of anabolism, catabolism, and immunity. J Int Soc Sports Nutr 2007;4:18.
8. Nieman DC. Immunonutrition support for athletes. Nutr Rev 2008;66(6):310–20.
9. Nieman DC, Peters EM, Henson DA, et al. Influence of vitamin C supplementation on cytokine changes following an ultramarathon. J Interferon Cytokine Res 2000; 20:1029–35.
10. Peterson EW, Ostrowski K, Ibfel T, et al. Effect of vitamin supplementation on cytokine response and on muscle damage after strenuous exercise. Am J Physiol Cell Physiol 2002;280:C1570–5.
11. Reynolds KA, Watt PM, Boone SA, et al. Occurrence of bacteria and biochemical markers on public surfaces. Int J Environ Health Res 2005;15(3):225–34.
12. Kaiser AB, Kernodle DS, Barg NL, et al. Influence of preoperative showers on staphylococcal skin colonization: a comparative trial of antiseptic skin cleaners. Ann Thorac Surg 1988;45(1):35–8.
13. Woodwell DA, Cherry DK. National ambulatory medical care survey: 2002 summary. Adv Data 2004;346:1–44.
14. Heikkinen T, Jarvinen A. The common cold. Lancet 2003;361:51–9.
15. Arroll B, Kenealy T. Antibiotics for the common cold and acute purulent rhinitis. Cochrane Database Syst Rev 2005;(3):CD000247.
16. Fahey T, Stocks N, Thomas T. Systematic review of the treatment of upper respiratory tract infection. Arch Dis Child 1998;79:225–30.
17. Simasek M, Bladino D. Treatment of the common cold. Am Fam Physician 2007; 75(4):515–20.
18. Linde K, Barrett B, Wolkart K, et al. *Echinacea* for preventing and treating the common cold. Cochrane Database Syst Rev 2006;(1):CD000530.
19. Yale SH, Liu K. *Echinacea purpurea* therapy for the treatment of the common cold: a randomized double-blind, placebo-controlled clinical trial. Arch Intern Med 2004;164:1237–41.
20. Turner RB, Bauer R, Woelkart K, et al. An evaluation of *Echinacea angustifolia* in experimental rhinovirus infections. N Engl J Med 2005;353:341–8.
21. Marchall I. Zinc for the common cold. Cochrane Database Syst Rev 1999;(2):CD001364.
22. Schroeder K, Fahey T. Over-the-counter medications for acute cough in children and adults in ambulatory settings. Cochrane Database Syst Rev 2004;(4):CD001831.
23. Irwin RS, Baumann MH, Bolser DC, et al. American College of Chest Physicians. Diagnosis and management of cough executive summary: ACCP evidence-based clinical practice guidelines. Chest 2006;129(Suppl 1):1S–23S.
24. Sutter AI, Lemiengre M, Campbell H, et al. Antihistamines for the common cold. Cochrane Database Syst Rev 2003;(3):CD001267.
25. Cantu C, Arauz A, Bonilla L, et al. Stroke associated with sympathomimetics contained in over-the-counter cough and cold drugs. Stroke 2003;34:1667–72.
26. Hentry DC, Moller DJ, Adelglass J, et al. Comparison of sparfloxacin and clarithromycin in the treatment of acute bacterial maxillary sinusitis. Sparfloxacin Multicenter AMS Study Group. Clin Ther 1999;21:340–52.
27. Low DE, Desrosiers M, McSherry J, et al. A practical guide for the diagnosis and treatment of acute sinusitis. CMAJ 1997;156(Suppl 6):S1–14.

28. Hickner JM, Bartlett JG, Besser RE, et al. Principles of appropriate antibiotic use for acute rhinosinusitis in adults: background. Ann Intern Med 2001;132(6):498–505.
29. Ah-See K. Sinusitus (acute). Clin Evid (Online) 2004;11:129–30.
30. Vincent MT, Celestin N, Hussain AN. Pharyngitis. Am Fam Physician 2004;69: 1465–70.
31. McIsaac WJ, Goel V, To T. The validity of a sore throat score in family practice. CMAJ 2000;163:811–5.
32. Mayes T, Pichichero ME. Are follow-up throat cultures necessary when rapid antigen detection tests are negative for group A streptococci? Clin Pediatr (Phila) 2001;40:191–5.
33. Bisno AL. Acute pharyngitis. N Engl J Med 2001;344:204–11.
34. Evans A, Niederman J. Epstein-Barr virus. Viral infections of human epidemiology and control. New York: Plenum Publishing; 1989. p. 265.
35. Rea TD, Russo JE, Katon W, et al. Prospective study of the natural history of infectious mononucleosis caused by Epstein-Barr virus. J Am Board Fam Pract 2001; 13:234–42.
36. Aldrete JS. Spontaneous rupture of the spleen in patients with infectious mononucleosis. Mayo Clin Proc 1992;67:910–2.
37. File TM. Community-acquired pneumonia. Lancet 2003;362:1991–2001.
38. Mandell LA, Bartlett JG, Dowell SF, et al. Infectious Diseases Society of America. Update of practice guidelines for the management of community-acquired pneumonia in immunocompetent adults. Clin Infect Dis 2003;37:1405–33.
39. Gonzales R, Sande MA. Uncomplicated acute bronchitis. Ann Intern Med 2000; 133:981–91.
40. Blinkhorn RJ Jr. Upper respiratory tract infections. In: Baum GL, editor. Textbook of pulmonary diseases. 6th edition. Philadelphia: Lippincott-Raven; 1998. p. 493–502.
41. Irwin RS, Curley FJ, Bennett FM. Appropriate use of antitussives and protussives. A practical review. Drugs 1993;46:80–91.
42. Hueston WJ. Albuterol delivered by metered-dose inhaler to treat acute bronchitis. J Fam Pract 1994;39:437–40.
43. Tingle LE, Molina D, Calvert CW. Acute pericarditis. Am Fam Physician 2007; 76(10):1509–14.
44. Spodick DH. Acute pericarditis: current concepts and practice. JAMA 2003;289: 1150–3.
45. Spodick DH. Pericardial diseases. In: Braunwald E, Zipes DP, Libby P, editors. Heart disease, a textbook of cardiovascular medicine. 6th edition. Philadelphia: WB Saunders; 2001. p. 1823–76.
46. Maisch B, Seferovic PM, Ristic AD, et al. for the Task Force on the Diagnosis and Management of Pericardial Diseases of the European Society of Cardiology. Guidelines on the diagnosis and management of pericardial diseases executive summary. Eur Heart J 2004;25:587–610.
47. Wynne J, Braunwald E. The cardiomyopathies and myocarditides. In: Braunwald E, Fauci A, Kasper D, editors. Harrison's principles of internal medicine. 15th edition. New York: McGraw Hill; 2001. p. 1359–65.
48. Puranic R, Chow CK, Duflou JA. Sudden death in the young. Heart Rhythm 2005; 2(12):1277–82.
49. Durakovic Z, Durakovic M, Skavic J. Myopericarditis and sudden cardiac death due to physical exercise in male athletes. Coll Antropol 2008;32(2):399–401.
50. Martin AG, Koboyashi GS. Superficial fungal infection: dermatophytosis, tinea nigra, piedra. In: Freedberg IM, et al, editors. 5th edition, Fitzpatrick's dermatology in general medicine, vol. 2. New York: McGraw-Hill; 1999. p. 2337–57.

51. Adams BB. Tinea corporis gladitorum. J Am Acad Dermatol 2002;47(2): 286–90.
52. Hainer BL. Dermatophyte infections. Am Fam Physician 2003;67:101–8.
53. Cobbold RJ, Macdonald A. Molluscum contagiosum as a sexually transmitted disease. Practitioner 1970;204:416–9.
54. Schwartz JJ, Myskowski PL. Molluscum contagiosum in patients with human immunodeficiency virus infection. A review of twenty-seven patients. J Am Acad Dermatol 1992;27:583–8.
55. Buller RM, Plumbo GJ. Poxvirus pathogenesis. Microbiol Rev 1991;55:80–122.
56. Ashcraft KA, Hunzeker J, Bonneau RH. Psychological stress impairs the local CD8+ T cell response to mucosal HSV-1 infection and allows for increased pathogenicity via a glucocorticoid receptor mediated mechanism. Psychoneuroendocrinology 2008;33(7):951–63 Epub 2008 Jul 25.
57. Brian B. Adams viral skin infections. In: Adams BB, editor. Sports dermatology. Springer; 2006. p. 35–46.
58. Nerukar LS, West F, May M, et al. Survival of herpes simplex virus in water specimens collected from hot tubs in spa facilities and on plastic surfaces. JAMA 1983;250:3081–3.
59. Ichihashi M, Nagai H, Matsunaga K. Sunlight is an important causative factor of recurrent herpes simplex. Cutis 2004;74(Suppl 5):14–8.
60. Holland EJ, Nahanti RL, Belongia EA, et al. Ocular involvement in an outbreak of herpes gladiatorum. Am J Ophthalmol 1992;114:680–4.
61. White WB, Grant-Kels JM. Transmission of herpes simplex virus type 1 infection in rugby players. JAMA 1984;252:533–5.
62. Salgado CD, Farr BM, Calfee DP. Community acquired methicillin-resistant *Staphylococcus aureus*: a meta-analysis of prevalence and risk factors. Clin Infect Dis 2003;36:131–9.
63. Brian B. Adams bacterial skin infections. In: Adams BB, editor. Sports dermatology. Springer; 2006. p. 3–34.
64. Nessel L. Florida fighter learns of MRSA infection after MMA bout. Florida Today February 21, 2009.
65. Kazakova SV, Hagemen JC, Matava M, et al. A clone of methicillin-resistant *Staphylococcus aureus* among professional football players. N Engl J Med 2005;352(5):468–75.
66. Bartlett PC, Martin RJ, Cahill BR. Furunculosis in a high school football team. Am J Sports Med 1982;10:371–4.
67. Sedgewick PE, Dexter WW, Smith CT. Bacterial dermatosis in sports. Clin Sports Med 2007;26:383–96.
68. Alcena V. Boxing and the transmission of HIV. N Y State J Med 1988;88(7):392.
69. Drotman DP. Professional boxing, bleeding and HIV testing. JAMA 1996;276(3): 193.
70. Centers for Disease Control and Prevention, national prevention information network. Available at: www.cdc.gov/hiv/resources. Accessed February 3, 2009.
71. Nattiv A, Puffer JC. Lifestyles and health risks of collegiate athletes. J Fam Pract 1991;33:585–90.
72. Sklarek HM, Mantovani RP, Erens E, et al. AIDS in a bodybuilder using anabolic steroids. N Engl J Med 1984;311:1701.
73. Torre D, Sampietro C, Ferraro G, et al. Transmission of HIV-1 infection via sports injury. Lancet 1990;335:1105.
74. O'Farrell N, Tovey SJ, Morgan-Capner P. Transmission of HIV-1 infection after a fight. Lancet 1992;339:246.

75. Ippolito G, Del Poggio P, Arici C. Transmission of zidovudine-resistant HIV during a bloody fight. JAMA 1992;272:433–4.
76. Perlmutter BL, Glaser JB, Oyugi SO. How to recognize and treat acute HIV syndrome. Am Fam Physician 1999;60:535–46.
77. Jordan BD. Aids and boxing. In: Jordan B, editor. Medical aspects of boxing. Boca Raton (FL): CRC Press; 2000. p. 317–22.
78. Souza PM, Jacob-Filho W, Santarém JM, et al. Progressive resistance training in elderly HIV positive patients: does it work? Clinics (Sau Paulo) 2008;63(5): 619–24.
79. Domingo hit with hepatitis B, Rocha fight called off. Available at: Boxingscene. com. Accessed November 21, 2008.
80. Bunce S. Boxing: skelton has the bulk and skill to shock Chagaev. Available at: independentNewsandMedia.com. Accessed January 19, 2008.
81. Lin KW, Kirchner JT. Hepatitis B. Am Fam Physician 2004;69:76.
82. Pediatrics Committee on Sports Medicine and Fitness. Human immunodeficiency virus and other blood-borne viral pathogens in the athletic setting. Pediatrics 1999;104:1400–3.
83. Parana R, Lyra L, Trepo C. Intravenous vitamin complexes used in sporting activities and transmission of HCV in Brazil. Am J Gastroenterol 1999;94:857–8.

# Brain Injury in Boxing

Barry D. Jordan, MD, MPH, FACSM[a,b,c,*]

**KEYWORDS**
- Acute traumatic brain injury • Chronic traumatic brain injury
- Sports concussion • Boxing injuries • Dementia pugilistica
- Alzheimer's disease • Second impact syndrome

Traumatic brain injury (TBI) is a common consequence of boxing. Accordingly, an understanding of TBI as it pertains to boxing is essential. Acute traumatic brain injury (ATBI), the second impact syndrome (SIS), and chronic traumatic brain injury (CTBI) may all be encountered in boxing. The epidemiology, clinical presentation, diagnosis, pathology, pathophysiology, management, and prevention of these neurologic syndromes are discussed.

## ACUTE TRAUMATIC BRAIN INJURY

ATBI is the immediate neurologic result of direct trauma to the head. Various acute traumatic injuries to the brain can be encountered in sports (**Box 1**). The most common type of ATBI encountered in boxing is cerebral concussion; however, more moderate to severe brain injuries such as subdural hematoma (SDH), cerebral contusion (CC), intracerebral hemorrhage (ICH), epidural hematoma (EDH), or diffuse axonal injury (DAI) may uncommonly be experienced by the combatant. Penetrating brain injuries and skull fractures are seldom encountered in boxing.

### Epidemiology

The frequency of ATBI in amateur boxing is low. Blonstein and Clarke[1] assessed boxing injuries in amateur boxers over a 7-month period and found that only 29 boxers (0.58%) were severely concussed or knocked out more than once. Injury reports from the 1981 and 1982 USA National Amateur Boxing Championships noted that 48 of 547 bouts (8.7%) were stopped because of knockouts (KOs) or blows to the head.[2] This yielded a rate of 4.38 head injuries per 100 personal exposures. In amateur boxing in Ireland, Porter and O'Brien[3] observed 33 cerebral concussions in 281 bouts or 562 personal exposures, yielding 5.87 concussions per 100 personal exposures.

---

[a] Brain Injury Program, Burke Rehabilitation Hospital, 785 Mamaroneck Avenue, White Plains, NY 10603, USA
[b] Department of Neurology, Weill Medical College of Cornell University, New York, NY, USA
[c] New York State Athletic Commission, New York, NY, USA
* Brain Injury Program, Burke Rehabilitation Hospital, 785 Mamaroneck Avenue, White Plains, NY 10603, USA
E-mail address: bjordan@burke.org

Clin Sports Med 28 (2009) 561–578
doi:10.1016/j.csm.2009.07.005
0278-5919/09/$ – see front matter © 2009 Elsevier Inc. All rights reserved.

---

**Box 1**
**Pathologic classification of acute traumatic brain injury in sports**

- Diffuse brain injury
  - Cerebral concussion
  - Diffuse axonal injury
- Focal brain injury
  - Epidural hematoma
  - Subdural hematoma
  - Cerebral contusion
  - Intracerebral hemorrhage
  - Subarachnoid hemorrhage
  - Intraventricular hemorrhage
- Skull fracture
- Penetrating brain injury

---

Jordan and colleagues[4] reviewed all boxing injuries sustained by amateur boxers at the United States Olympic Training Center (USOTC) during a 10-year period. Among the total of 477 injuries, only 29 (6.5%) were brain injuries. In another survey of amateur boxers in Denmark, 5.7% to 7.8% of boxing competitions resulted in a KO and 0.8% to 5.4% of the bouts were terminated because the referee stopped the contest secondary to head blows (RSCH).[5] Welch and colleagues[6] conducted a survey of boxing injuries that occurred during an institutional boxing program at the US Military Academy (SMA) in West Point, New York, over a 2-year period. Although approximately 2100 cadets received boxing instruction, only 22 cases of blunt head trauma were reported, none of which resulted in neurologic deficits.

The frequency of ATBI among professional boxers tends to be higher than among amateur boxers. Jordan and Campbell[7] reviewed all acute boxing injuries among professional boxers in New York State from August, 1982 to July, 1984. During this 2-year period there were 3110 rounds fought and 376 injuries, of which 262 were head injuries, yielding a frequency of 0.8 head injuries per 10 rounds fought and 2.9 injuries per 10 boxers. In a survey of a representative sample of active professional boxers in New York State, the prevalence of a self-reported technical knockout (TKO) or KO was 42% (143 boxers).[8] Also observed in New York State was a tendency for TKOs or KOs to occur in the earlier rounds. In 1 year, 122 of 189 bouts (65%) resulted in a TKO or KO and 80% of these occurred within the first 3 rounds.[9] A review of professional boxing injuries in Victoria, Australia, from August, 1985 to August, 2001 reported a total of 107 injuries among a total of 427 boxers. In this survey concussions comprised 15.9% of all injuries.[10]

Evidence suggests that medical injuries among female boxers may occur less frequently than those in male boxers. A medical survey of boxing injuries among amateur and professional female boxers in Italy from 2002 to 2003 indicates that ATBIs among female contestants are rare.[11] Bledsoe and colleagues conducted a review of professional boxing injuries in the state of Nevada from September, 2001 to March, 2003. The overall incidence rate of injury was 17.1 per 100 boxer-matches or 3.4 per 100 boxer-rounds.[12] Male boxers were significantly more likely than female boxers to receive injuries (3.6 versus 1.2 per 100 boxer-rounds).

Furthermore, male boxing matches resulted in TKO and KO more frequently than female matches. The incidence rate of injury among those boxers who lost their bout was nearly twice the rate of the winning boxers.

### Clinical Presentation

Common signs and symptoms of ATBI, which may have cognitive, behavioral or neurophysical features, are presented in **Box 2**. Cognitive impairment after a boxing match may include problems with attention, planning, and memory.[13] An amnestic period with confusion appears to be characteristic of many KOs,[14] but amnesia can

---

**Box 2**
**Common signs and symptoms of ATBI**

*Cognitive features*
- Decreased speed of information processing
- Disorientation
- Unawareness
- Confusion
- Amnesia/memory impairment
- Impaired concentration
- Loss of consciousness
- Fogginess

*Behavioral features*
- Sleep disturbance
- Irritability
- Emotional ability
- Nervousness/anxiety
- Psychomotor retardation
- Apathy
- Fatigue
- Easily distracted

*Physical features*
- Headache
- Dizziness/vertigo
- Nausea
- Vacant stare
- Impaired playing ability
- Gait unsteadiness/loss of balance
- Impaired coordination
- Diplopia
- Photophobia
- Hyperacusis
- Concussive convulsion/impact seizure

occur without a KO and should be regarded as evidence of serious injury.[15] Blonstein and Clarke[1] described a boxer who won a decision but was amnesic for the entire fight despite not being knocked out. Retrograde and anterograde amnesia have been described in boxing.[16]

In addition to cognitive impairment, various other neurologic symptoms may be encountered in boxing. Sercl and Jaros[17] analyzed the acute neurologic findings in 427 boxers involved in 1165 matches. A total of 336 (79%) boxers had clinical abnormalities that resolved within several minutes and 91 (21%) had neurologic symptoms lasting up to 24 hours. The most common clinical findings were derangement of muscular tone (380 cases), followed by cerebellar and vestibular signs (319 cases) and pyramidal symptoms (253 cases). Other findings included unconsciousness (112 cases), extrapyramidal signs (191 cases), and general muscular weakness (142 cases). Cranial nerve lesions were exceedingly rare (7 cases).

The ascertainment of a concussion during a boxing match may be difficult because most concussions in boxing are not associated with loss of consciousness (LOC), and boxers who sustain a TKO or KO secondary to blows to the head may or may not experience concussion. The authors conducted an analysis of 316 TKO/KOs secondary to head blows among professional boxers in New York State from January, 1996 to December, 2001. Most boxers experiencing a TKO/KO did not exhibit LOC (76%). Sixty (19%) boxers experienced LOC that was witnessed by the ringside physician (see **Table 1**). Among those with LOC, 53 (17%) exhibited a brief LOC that resolved in less than 1 minute. Only 7 (2%) boxers exhibited LOC lasting longer than 1 minute. None of the boxers exhibited LOC lasting 5 minutes or longer. The duration of LOC was not recorded in 17 (5%) boxers. Most of the boxers experienced a rapid recovery (ie, no complaint of neurologic symptoms or abnormalities on gross neurologic examination). A total of 269 (85%) boxers recovered neurologic function within 5 minutes. Fifteen (5%) boxers required more than 5 minutes to recover. The duration of time required for recovery of function was not recorded in 32 (10%). Eleven (3%) boxers were transferred to hospital for further neurologic evaluation. Nine of these boxers exhibited LOC and had delayed recovery of function (ie, longer than 5 minutes to regain neurologic function). Two boxers who required further neurologic evaluation and did not exhibit LOC had persistent neurologic symptoms and took longer than 5 minutes to recover function. Among the 316 TKO/KOs, 2 were considered serious. One boxer died of a subdural hematoma and the other had a severe concussion that ended his career.

**Table 1**
**Clinical characteristics of 316 acute traumatic brain injuries in New York State**

| Loss of Consciousness | Number (%) |
| --- | --- |
| None | 239 (76) |
| <1 min | 53 (17) |
| >1 min | 7 (2) |
| Not recorded | 17 (5) |
| Total | 316 |
| **Time to Recovery** | **Number (%)** |
| <5 min | 269 (85) |
| >5 min | 15 (5) |
| Not recorded | 32 (10) |
| Total | 316 |

Another survey of clinical characteristics of 187 boxers licensed to box professionally in New York State, who were medically suspended as a consequence of a TKO/KO from 2002 to 2005, is presented in **Table 2**. Of the 187 professional boxers, 142 (75.9%) lost their bout by TKO and 158 (84.5%) had no period of LOC. Most of the boxers (179) (95.7%) were able to leave the ring unassisted after their defeat. Ten (5.3%) boxers required more than 5 minutes to recover full neurologic functioning. Neurologic symptoms exhibited by boxers who experienced a TKO/KO are presented in **Table 3**. Gait difficulties were observed in 40.6% of the boxers. Twenty-six boxers (20.3%) were confused or not fully oriented to person, place, and time. Eleven (8.5%) boxers responded slowly to questions, and balance problems were recognized in 9 boxers (7%). The Glasgow Coma Scale (GCS) score (**Table 4**) was also used to assess neurologic function among these 187 professional boxers who experienced a TKO or KO and who were classified mild, moderate, or severe (**Table 5**). Of the professional boxers examined, 96% were classified as mild TBI (ie, GCS score 13–15) (**Table 6**); 89.3% (167 boxers) scored 15 points and 8.6% (16 boxers) scored 14 points. Only 2 (1.1%) boxers scored in the severe range, with 3 points each. One boxer with an injury of moderate severity had a GCS score of 11. These findings suggest that the GCS may be insensitive to assessing neurologic function in boxers who experience a TKO or KO.

## Diagnosis

ATBI is diagnosed by a comprehensive neurologic examination documenting the neurologic signs and symptoms mentioned earlier in this discussion following a direct or indirect mechanical force to the brain. The GCS is an insensitive tool for the assessment of concussion in boxing; almost 90% of boxers sustaining a TKO/KO had a normal score (GCS score = 15). However, the GCS score does afford the opportunity to document those boxers with moderate or severe brain injury and provide guidelines for the proper emergency triage (see section on management of ATBI).

In addition to the neurologic examination, neuropsychological testing and neuroimaging may be indicated in the assessment of ATBI associated with boxing. Neuropsychological testing can be used to determine the extent of cognitive and behavioral impairment following ATBI and can be used to help document recovery following TBI in individuals with baseline testing. Neuroimaging in ATBI is indicated in boxers with prolonged or severe symptoms following a concussion or in boxers with moderate (GCS score 9–12) or severe (GCS score 3–8) TBI.

## Pathology

Concussion is the most common ATBI encountered in boxing and is not typically associated with any gross pathologic changes. Microscopically, animal studies

**Table 2**
**Characteristics of 187 professional boxers according to accident report**

| Variables | Number of Boxers (%) | Number of Boxers (%) |
|---|---|---|
| LOC Y/N | 28 (15.0) | 159 (85.0%) |
| TKO/KO | 142 (75.9) | 31 (16.6) |
| LR Y/N | 179 (95.7) | 6 (3.2) |
| TTR <5/>5 | 150 (80.20) | 10 (5.3) |
| NS Y/N | 94 (50.3) | 93 (49.7) |

*Abbreviations:* LOC, loss of consciousness; LR, leave ring unassisted; NS, neurologic symptoms; TTR, time to recover full neurologic functioning in minutes; Y/N, yes/no.

**Table 3**
**Neurologic symptoms shown by boxer post bout**

| | |
|---|---|
| Difficulty gait | 52 (40.6) |
| Confusion | 26 (20.3) |
| Slow speech | 11 (8.5) |
| Balance problems | 9 (7.0) |
| Dazed | 8 (6.2) |
| Decreased coordination | 6 (4.6) |
| Dizziness | 5 (3.9) |
| Headache | 4 (3.1) |
| LOC | 3 (2.3) |
| Memory problems | 1 (0.7) |
| Weakness arm/leg | 1 (0.7) |
| Slurred speech | 1 (0.7) |
| Agitation | 1 (0.7) |

suggest that chromatolysis can occur after concussion.[18] However, when extrapolating to humans, the severity of the head trauma experienced by the experimental animals in these investigations may be more significant than what is typically encountered in boxing. In human studies, Oppenheimer[19] observed microscopic changes such as axonal retraction balls and myelin destruction in the setting of microglial clusters after a concussion. However, the contribution of anoxia to these neuropathologic changes was difficult to assess. Accordingly, whether the uncomplicated concussion in boxing (ie, without anoxia or reduced cerebral perfusion) results in structural damage remains to be determined.

Although uncommon, acute catastrophic pathologic lesions such as diffuse axonal injury, subdural hematoma, epidural hematoma, cerebral contusion, intracerebral hemorrhage, injury to the carotid, and subarachnoid hemorrhage may be encountered in boxers.[20,21]

**Table 4**
**Glasgow coma score**

| Response | | Score |
|---|---|---|
| Verbal | None | 1 |
| | Incomprehensible sounds | 2 |
| | Inappropriate words | 3 |
| | Confused | 4 |
| | Oriented | 5 |
| Eye opening | None | 1 |
| | To pain | 2 |
| | To speech | 3 |
| | Spontaneously | 4 |
| Motor | None | 1 |
| | Abnormal extension | 2 |
| | Abnormal flexion | 3 |
| | Withdraws | 4 |
| | Localizes | 5 |
| | Obeys | 6 |

| Table 5 | |
|---|---|
| **Clinical classification of traumatic brain injury according to the Glasgow Coma Scale score** | |
| Mild | 13–15 |
| Moderate | 9–12 |
| Severe | 3–8 |

## Pathophysiology

The concussive properties of a boxer's punch are related to the manner in which the punch is delivered, and how the mechanical forces are transferred and absorbed through the intracranial cavity. Blows thrown from the shoulder, such as the round-house or the hook, tend to deliver more force than the straightforward jab. An analysis of blows delivered by Olympic boxers to the head of an instrumented Hybrid III dummy noted that the hook produced the greatest change in hand velocity and generated the greatest punch force compared with straight punches and uppercuts.[22] The force transmitted by a punch is directly proportional to the mass of the glove and the velocity of the swing, and is inversely proportional to the total mass opposing the punch.[23] Punch force has been observed to be greater among heavier boxers secondary to a higher effective mass of the punch.[24]

The essential feature of a concussive force is that it is sufficient to accelerate the skull. Rotational (angular) acceleration, linear (translational) acceleration, and impact deceleration can all play a role in the development of acute cerebral injury.[20] Angular acceleration occurs when a punch causes a rotational movement of the skull that can potentially stretch and tear cerebral blood vessels. Subdural hematomas typically result from tearing of the bridging veins secondary to rotational acceleration. Rotational acceleration is also responsible for diffuse axonal injury. Linear acceleration occurs with blows directly to the face, which can propel the skull in an anterior to posterior direction and may result in gliding contusions. Impact deceleration, which occurs when the head strikes the mat after a boxer is knocked to the canvas, can potentially cause a second traumatic brain injury.[20]

Trauma to the brain initiates a pathophysiologic cascade of molecular and neurometabolic events (**Box 3**). These include neurotransmitter changes, ionic alterations, metabolic dysfunction, apoptosis, and inflammatory processes. A full discussion of these events is beyond the scope of this article; however, readers are referred to the text of Miller and Hayes for a comprehensive review.[25]

## Management

The treatment of ATBI is dependent on the type and severity of the injury. Because most acute brain injuries are concussions, the typical management requires

| Table 6 | |
|---|---|
| **Postbout Glasgow Coma Scale score of 187 knocked-out boxers** | |
| **Postbout GCS Score (Points)** | **Number of Boxers (%)** |
| 15 | 167 (89.3) |
| 14 | 16 (8.6) |
| 13 | 1 (0.5) |
| 11 | 1 (0.5) |
| 3 | 2 (1.1) |

---

**Box 3**
**Molecular mechanisms in the pathophysiology of traumatic brain injury**

Glutamate toxicity

Ionic alterations

Inflammatory responses

Cholinergic dysfunction

Growth factor alterations

Apoptosis

Calpain/caspase activation

Mitochondrial dysfunction

Free radical formation and peroxidation

---

observation because these injuries are usually self-limited. However, it becomes imperative for the clinician to be aware of more potentially dangerous injuries to the central nervous system (CNS) (**Box 4**). Indicators of more ominous neurologic injuries include GCS score 3 to 12, prolonged LOC (longer than a few minutes), focal neurologic signs, seizures, or persistent postconcussive symptoms (longer than 24 hours). Any boxer suspected of experiencing an acute focal TBI during a competitive bout should be immediately transported by ambulance to the nearest hospital equipped with proper neuroradiological and neurosurgical services. Any boxer who experiences persistent postconcussive symptoms should be properly evaluated and not allowed to return to competition until they are asymptomatic. Traditional guidelines used for the return to competition after concussion in sports[26,27] have not been routinely used in boxing. In boxing, the recommendations for rest or inactivity after a concussion vary from boxing jurisdiction and whether it is amateur or professional boxing. However, return to competition following a concussion should follow the same recommendations as outlined by the 2008 Zurich Consensus Statement on Concussion in Sport.[28]

### Prevention

ATBI in boxing is virtually impossible to eliminate. However, the mainstay of prevention should be to minimize the severity of the ATBI. This goal could be accomplished by conducting prefight examinations to identify individuals predisposed to acute catastrophic brain injury. In addition to the prefight neurologic examination, neuroimaging

---

**Box 4**
**Indication for neurologic evaluation following aTBI in boxing**

GCS score of 3–12

Loss of consciousness associated with delayed recovery of function

Persistent neurologic symptoms lasting longer than 24 hours

Focal neurologic deficits (ie, hemiparesis, hemisensory loss, aphasia or unilateral hyperreflexia

Seizures (focal or generalized), not including impact seizures

Clinical evidence of skull fracture (ie, Battle's sign, raccoon eyes, or cranial nerve palsies)

or neuropsychological testing may be useful in protecting the health and safety of the boxer.

Surveillance prebout neuroimaging can be invaluable in detecting preexisting brain lesions that may dispose a boxer to catastrophic brain injury. Neuropsychological testing can identify those boxers who are still experiencing cognitive impairment following a concussion. If possible baseline neuropsychological testing should be performed so that if the boxer sustains a concussion follow-up neuropsychological testing can be performed to ensure that the boxer has recovered cognitively.

In addition to performing the prefight examination, there should be qualified medical personnel at the ringside (and an ambulance), who can provide medical assistance to the injured boxer. After a competition, all boxers should be briefly examined by the ringside physician. The referee is also instrumental in increasing medical safety in the ring. A qualified referee should be able to identify a boxer who is experiencing a concussion and terminate the bout before more neurologic injury can occur. The entire boxing community (including the trainer and the promoter) should work together to increase medical safety in boxing.[29]

## SECOND IMPACT SYNDROME

The second impact syndrome (SIS) represents an exaggerated, commonly fatal response to a second concussion while an athlete is symptomatic from an earlier concussion.[30–32] SIS was initially described by Saunders and Harbaugh[30] and has been noted primarily in tackle football. However, SIS can be anticipated in any contact sport and has been described in boxing.[31]

### Epidemiology

The exact frequency of SIS in sports is unknown but it is believed to be uncommon. Risk factors for SIS have not been clearly established.[32] However, any boxer or athlete who participates in a contact/collision sport while symptomatic from a concussion seems to be at increased risk of SIS. In boxing, SIS may occur in a tournament setting when a boxer competes more than once over a selected time period (typically a few days to a week), or it may occur less frequently within a given bout associated with multiple concussive blows.

### Clinical Presentation

Clinically, the athlete will experience a mild traumatic brain injury (most typically a concussion) followed by persistent postconcussive symptoms, which may include cognitive, behavioral, or neurophysical symptoms (see **Box 2**). While symptomatic from the first brain injury the athlete returns to participation and sustains a second traumatic brain injury, which may be minor and may not even involve direct head trauma.[31] After sustaining this second impact, the athlete may collapse into a coma with rapid brainstem compromise, respiratory failure, and possible death.[31]

### Diagnosis

According to McCrory and Berkovic[32] the following clinical criteria need to be fulfilled for the definitive diagnosis of SIS:

a. Medical review after a witnessed first impact
b. Documentation of ongoing symptoms following the first impact up to the time of the second impact
c. Witnessed second head impact with a subsequent rapid cerebral deterioration

d. Neuropathologic or neuroimaging evidence of cerebral swelling without significant intracranial hematoma or other cause for edema

In boxing, the diagnosis of SIS may be difficult if a boxer sustains an unrecognized concussion during a bout and then sustains a second concussion during the same competition while symptomatic from the initial concussion. In this scenario, SIS may be suspected in the boxer who collapses in the ring after a blow to the head during competition or sparring and exhibits massive cerebral edema on neuroimaging without other significant neuropathology.

### Pathology/Pathophysiology

The postmortem hallmark of SIS is massive cerebral edema. Although subdural hematomas may be encountered, they tend to be small and of no clinical significance.[31] The pathophysiologic mechanism of SIS seems to be loss of vasomotor autoregulation, leading to excessive hyperemia or cerebrovascular engorgement, resulting in massive cerebral swelling and brain herniation. Animal studies suggest that repetitive brain injury results in a breakdown of the blood-brain barrier (BBB) and that the brain remains vulnerable for a period of time and susceptible to the effects of a second concussive blow.[33]

### Management

The management of a boxer experiencing SIS requires emergent medical and neurologic attention because of associated morbidity and mortality. More typically these injuries tend to be moderate or severe brain injuries (ie, GCS score 3–12). Any boxer suspected of experiencing SIS should be transferred immediately to a medical facility that is equipped with neuroradiological and neurosurgical services.

### Prevention

In view of the high mortality and morbidity associated with SIS, the prevention of this syndrome becomes paramount. The mainstay of preventive measures relies on the proper evaluation of the athlete who sustains an ATBI. Any athlete who sustains an ATBI should undergo a detailed neurologic evaluation to determine the severity of the injury. In cases of cerebral concussion the athlete should not be allowed to return to competition unless they are asymptomatic for a period of time and neurologic and cognitive function has returned to normal.[28] Neuropsychological testing may provide additional insight as to whether a boxer has recovered full neurocognitive function. However, this is best implemented if there is a preexisting baseline for comparison. The restriction of the symptomatic boxer from participating in sparring or competition should minimize the occurrence of SIS.

### CHRONIC TRAUMATIC BRAIN INJURY

Chronic traumatic brain injury (CTBI), also known as dementia pugilistica, chronic traumatic encephalopathy, chronic neurologic injury, or the "punch drunk" syndrome, is the long-term cumulative neurologic consequence of repetitive concussive and subconcussive blows to the head. This syndrome was first described in the medical literature by Martland[34] in 1928, when he described a 38-year-old retired boxer with advanced parkinsonism, ataxia, pyramidal tract dysfunction, and behavioral changes. CTBI is typically delayed in onset and occurs after a long exposure to the sport, usually after a boxer retires or late in the boxer's career. As a result of this delayed onset, CTBI represents the most difficult safety challenge in modern-day boxing.

## Epidemiology

The true incidence and prevalence of CTBI in modern-era boxing is unknown. Among ex-professional boxers who were licensed by the British Board of Control for at least 3 years from 1929 to 1955, it has been estimated that the prevalence of CTBI is 17%, and the prevalence increases with increasing exposure to boxing.[35] However, it has been speculated that the risk of CTBI diminishes secondary to reduction in exposure to repetitive head trauma and increasing medical monitoring of boxers.[36] Strong objective evidence linking CTBI with amateur boxing is lacking.[37]

Putative and established risk factors for CTBI are presented in **Box 5**. Increased exposure probably represents the most important risk factor for CTBI. Documented risk factors for CTBI in boxing include later retirement (ie, more than 28 years of age), increased duration of career (ie, more than 10 years), and a greater number of bouts (ie, more than 150 bouts).[35] In a systematic review of observational studies in amateur boxing, CTBI does not seem to be strongly associated with CTBI. Clinical studies among professional boxers suggest that risk factors for the development of CTBI include poor performance (ie, second- or third-rate boxers), boxing style (ie, being a slugger, rather than a scientific, intelligent boxer), boxers who are notorious for their ability to take a punch, and being a professional boxer as opposed to amateur.[16] The age at examination also influenced the prevalence of CTBI. Boxers who were examined after the age of 50 years had a higher prevalence of CTBI than those examined before the age of 50 years.[35] Increasing sparring exposure may increase the risk of neurocognitive decline among professional boxers.[38] A history of a TKO or KO has also been reported to be associated with an abnormal computed tomographic (CT) scan of the brain.[8] In addition, progressive changes on CT scans have been noted in boxers who lose more than 10 bouts.[39]

Recent MRI surveillance studies of active boxers have found associations between boxing history and abnormalities on MRI. A review of brain MRI scans for boxers applying for licensure at the New York State Athletic Commission is presented in **Tables 7** and **8**. Boxers exhibiting a cavum septum pellucidum (CSP) (a common radiological finding among boxers with long exposure to boxing) on MRI tended to experience more losses, more TKO/KOs, and medical suspensions (see **Table 7**). Boxers with white-matter changes on MRI (which are nonspecific and potentially related to brain trauma) were also noted to have an increased frequency of losses (see **Table 8**). Orrison and colleagues[40] using high-field MRI to evaluate 100 unarmed

---

**Box 5**
**Putative and documented risk factors for chronic traumatic brain injury**

Total number of fights

Number of knockouts experienced

Number of losses

Duration of boxing career

Fight frequency

Age of retirement from boxing

Sparring exposure

Poor performance or skills

APOE e4 genotype

**Table 7**
Boxing history among boxers with and those without cavum septum pellucidum on brain MRI in New York State

| | With CSP (Positive) (n = 15) | Without CSP Negative (n = 127) | P Value |
|---|---|---|---|
| Age | 30.41 | 28.06 | 0.07 |
| Wins | 11.1 | 8.4 | 0.1 |
| Losses | 3.3 | 2.4 | 0.01 |
| Total bouts | 14.8 | 11.4 | 0.08 |
| Total rounds of fought | 62.9 | 54.9 | 0.07 |
| KO/TKO experienced | 1.5 | 0.8 | 0.02 |
| Duration of career (months) | 50.1 | 38.1 | 0.1 |
| Fights frequency (fights/y) | 5.51 | 4.27 | 0.1 |
| Suspensions | 1.3 | 0.7 | 0.003 |
| Spar rounds/wk | 17.3 | 14.9 | 0.4 |
| Weeks preparation for a bout | 6.0 | 6.6 | 0.5 |
| Weight loss (lb) before bout | 7.0 | 7.0 | 0.8 |
| Days rest before bout | 4.7 | 5.4 | 0.4 |

combatants (boxers and mixed martial artists) observed a statistical association between the number of bouts and increased lateral ventricular size. They also observed that longer careers were associated with the presence of dilated perivascular spaces and evidence suggestive of DAI. These findings indirectly support the hypothesis that poor performance or long exposure to boxing may increase the risk of cumulative boxing-related brain trauma.

### Clinical Presentation

In a comprehensive review of the neuropsychiatric aspects of boxing, Mendez[41] classified the clinical manifestations of CTBI into motor, cognitive, and psychiatric symptoms. Early signs of CTBI may include dysarthria, mild incoordination, tremor, and decreased complex attention. Psychiatric symptoms may include emotional lability and other mild behavioral disturbances such as euphoria or hypomania and increased irritability. Although it has been observed that the initial manifestations of CTBI are predominantly psychiatric or behavioral in nature,[42] it is the experience of the author that the behavioral and personality disturbances may be difficult to assess early in the disease, particularly when the examiner lacks knowledge of the boxer's premorbid personality. The second or moderate stage of CTBI is characterized by a progression of the motor, cognitive, or behavioral symptoms.[41] Motorically, boxers exhibit signs of parkinsonism or progressive difficulty in coordination and ambulation. Cognitive deficits include mild deficits in memory, attention, and executive function. Psychiatric manifestations may include inappropriate behavior, morbid jealousy, paranoia, and violent outbursts. The third or severe stage of CTBI is often referred to as dementia pugilistica.[41] During this phase of the disorder, the boxer exhibits significant motor dysfunction characterized by prominent pyramidal, extrapyramidal, or cerebellar symptoms. Cognitive dysfunction as evidenced by amnesia, executive-frontal lobe dysfunction, and psychomotor retardation may be observed. Behaviorally, boxers may exhibit disinhibition, violent outbursts, hypersexuality, and psychosis.[41]

**Table 8**
Boxing history among boxers with and those without white-matter changes on brain MRI in New York State

| | With White-Matter Changes (Abnormal) (n = 15) | Without White-Matter Changes (Normal) (n = 127) | P Value |
|---|---|---|---|
| Age | 29.74 | 28.14 | 0.2 |
| Wins | 11.7 | 8.3 | 0.4 |
| Losses | 4.7 | 2.3 | 0.03 |
| Total bouts | 17.1 | 11.1 | 0.4 |
| Total rounds fought | 85.1 | 52.3 | 0.3 |
| KO/TKO experienced | 1.7 | 0.8 | 0.2 |
| Durations of career (months) | 56.9 | 37.3 | 0.3 |
| Fight frequency (fights/y) | 4.11 | 4.44 | 0.8 |
| Suspensions | 0.7 | 0.7 | 0.6 |
| Spar rounds/wk | 11.6 | 15.5 | 0.1 |
| Weeks preparation for bout | 5.3 | 6.6 | 0.2 |
| Weight loss (lb) before bout | 6.5 | 7.0 | 0.6 |
| Days rest before bout | 6.0 | 5.3 | 0.98 |

## Diagnosis

In addition to a detailed neurologic examination documenting cognitive, behavioral, or motor impairments in a boxer, various neurodiagnostic tests have been used in the evaluation of the boxer with suspected CTBI. Structural neuroimaging demonstrates nonspecific findings in CTBI. Computed tomography (CT) and magnetic resonance imaging (MRI) may demonstrate brain atrophy with or without a CSD.[8,39,40,43–47] Diffusion tensor imaging (DTI) can document injury to the white-matter tracts among active boxers.[48]

The use of functional neuroimaging in boxing has been limited. Single photon emission computed tomography (SPECT) may exhibit perfusion deficits in boxers[49,50] that localize primarily to the frontal and temporal regions.[50] Positron emission tomography (PET) scanning may demonstrate hypometabolism in the bilateral posterior parietal lobes, bilateral frontal lobes, bilateral cerebellar hemispheres, and posterior cingulate gyrus[51] Some features noted on PET scanning share similar characteristic features consistent with Alzheimer disease (AD). **Fig. 1** shows biparietal and bitemporal hypometabolism on a PET scan of an aymptomatic 26-year-old boxer who had a normal MRI of the brain and whose APOE genotype was ε3/ε3. Magnetic resonance spectroscopy (MRS) provides a noninvasive means of identifying neurometabolic changes of the brain, indicating neuroinflammation.[52] The electroencephalogram (EEG) has a limited role in the evaluation of a boxer with CTBI. The EEG may be normal or may demonstrate focal or diffuse slowing.[35,53,54]

## Pathology

Pathologically, boxers with end-stage CTBI or full-blown dementia pugilistica may exhibit septal and hypothalamic anomalies, cerebellar changes, degeneration of the substantia nigra, and regional occurrence of Alzheimer's neurofibrillary tangles (NFTs).[55,56] Boxers may exhibit a fenestrated septal cavum, the floor of the hypothalamus may appear to be stretched, and the fornix and mammillary bodies may be

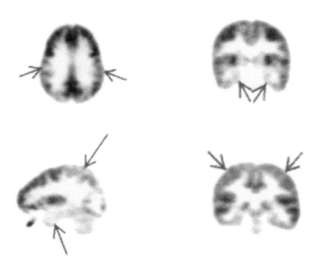

**Fig. 1.** Positron emission tomography scan of a 26-year-old asymptomatic boxer demonstrating biparietal and bitemporal hypometabolism similar to that seen in Alzheimer's disease.

atrophied. The cerebellum may demonstrate scarring of the folia in the region of the cerebellar tonsils, and there may be a reduction in the number of Purkinje cells on the inferior surface of the cerebellum. The substantia nigra may lack pigment, and nerve cells may become gliosed. NFTs primarily involving parts of the hippocampus and the medial temporal gray matter may also be encountered. NFTs are not typically accompanied by senile neuritic plaques but may be accompanied by diffuse amyloid plaques.[57,58] NFTs observed in boxers with CTBI are also immunoreactive for tau[58] and ubiquitin,[59] similar to those seen in AD. Another similarity that CTBI shares with AD is a significant reduction of choline acetyltransferase activity in the nucleus basalis of Meynert (nbM) and in several regions of the cerebral cortex.[60] Uryu and colleagues[61] in an animal model of TBI noted that TBI induces the rapid accumulation of key proteins that form pathologic aggregates in neurodegenerative disorders, such as AD.

### Pathophysiology

The pathophysiology of CTBI is unknown. However, any theory of the pathogenesis of CTBI must delineate the interactions between head trauma, NFT formation, amyloid deposition, central cholinergic function, and subsequent cognitive impairment. CTBI may share a similar pathogenic mechanism to that of AD.[57] Because CTBI seems to be primarily a tangle disease, any account of the pathophysiology of CTBI would have to consider the pathologic role of NFT formation. Amyloid metabolism and deposition may be involved in the pathophysiology of CTBI, however this needs to be further delineated. The role of the cholinergic system in the pathogenesis of CTBI remains to be determined. Animal studies indicate that concussive head injury has a profound effect on central cholinergic neurons.[62] Furthermore, the cholinergic system has been implicated in the pathophysiology of AD and is probably involved in the physiologic basis of learning and memory.[63] Accordingly, any theory of the pathogenesis of CTBI must delineate the interactions between head trauma, NFT formation, amyloid deposition, central cholinergic function, and subsequent cognitive impairment.

The role of apolipoprotein E (APOE) e4 allele in the development of CTBI also needs to be explored. Evidence suggests that the presence of the APOE e4 allele may promote the deposition of cerebral amyloid in individuals experiencing traumatic brain injury.[64] Mayeaux and colleagues[65] noted a 10-fold synergistic increased risk of AD in individuals with traumatic brain injury and the presence of APOE e4, whereas an addictive increased risk of AD in patients with head trauma and APOE e4 was observed by Katzman and colleagues.[66] Based on the author's observation of extensive parenchymal cerebral amyloid deposition and cerebral amyloid angiopathy in a demented boxer who harbored an APOE e4 allele,[67] the author conducted a study to determine whether APOE e4 is associated with CTBI.[56] In an analysis of 30 active and retired boxers, the author found that APOE e4 was associated with an increased severity of CTBI in high-exposure boxers (ie, boxers with more than 12 professional bouts). This finding suggests that there may be a genetic predisposition to the untoward effects of a long boxing career.[68]

## Management

A definitive treatment of CTBI has not been clearly established. In view of the pathologic similarities between CTBI and AD, standard treatments for the management of the cognitive and behavioral symptoms in AD may be employed in CTBI. However, the efficacy of these interventions has not been determined. Boxers with parkinsonian features may be treated with conventional dopaminergic agents used in Parkinson disease.

## Prevention

The mainstay of preventing CTBI in boxing is to limit exposure and identify those boxers who may be at increased risk of CTBI. Boxers who may be at increased risk of CTBI (see **Box 5**) should undergo more detailed neurodiagnostic testing such as MRI, SPECT, and neuropsychological testing. Whether APOE genotyping will prove useful in the prevention of CTBI remains to be determined, but it is a controversial topic.[69] Theoretically, boxers who are APOE e4 positive can be informed of the potential risks and followed more closely from the neurologic standpoint.

## SUMMARY

Acute and chronic TBI and SIS are major medical concerns in modern-day boxing. Despite the frequency of concussions in boxing, catastrophic ATBI is infrequent, and is minimized by pre- and postbout medical evaluations. The proper management of boxers with postconcussive symptoms will limit the frequency of SIS. CTBI, which shares many similarities with AD, represents the most significant public health concern in boxing. The identification of high-risk boxers who would be subjected to more detailed neurologic testing may help to lower the prevalence of CTBI. The role of genetic testing in preventing brain injury in boxing remains to be determined.

## ACKNOWLEDGMENTS

Special thanks to George M. Hanna, Ronald D. Howell, Nadyia Monday, Martin J. Kempa, and Karina Ortega-Verdejo for their assistance in the data collection and analysis of the medical records from the New York state Athletic Commission.

## REFERENCES

1. Blonstein JL, Clarke E. Further observations on the medical aspects of amateur boxing. Br Med J 1957;1:362–4.
2. Estwanik JJ, Boitano M, Ari N. Amateur boxing injuries at the 1981 and 1982 USA/ABF national championships. Phys Sports Med 1984;12:123–8.
3. Porter M, O'Brien. Incidence and severity of injuries resulting from amateur boxing in Ireland. Clin J Sport Med 1996;6:97–101.
4. Jordan BD, Voy RO, Stone J. Amateur boxing injuries at the United States Olympic Training Center. Phys Sports Med 1990;18(2):80–90.
5. Schmidt-Olsen S, Jensen SK, Mortensen V. Amateur boxing in Denmark: the effect of some preventive measures. Am J Sports Med 1990;18:98–100.
6. Welch MJ, Sitler M, Kroeten H. Boxing injuries from an instructional program. Phys Sports Med 1986;14:81–9.
7. Jordan BD, Campbell E. Acute boxing injuries among professional boxers in New York State: a two-year survey. Phys Sports Med 1988;16:87–91.
8. Jordan BD, Jahre C, Hauser WA, et al. CT of 338 active professional boxers. Radiology 1992;185:509–12.
9. Jordan BD. Professional boxing: experience of the New York State athletic commission. In: Cantu RC, editor. Boxing and medicine. Champaign (IL): Human Kinetics; 1995. p. 177–85.
10. Zazryn TR, Finch CF, McCrory PA. 16 year study of injuries to professional boxers in the state of Victoria, Australia. Br J Sports Med 2003;37:321–4.
11. Bianco M, Pannozzo A, Fabbricatore C, et al. Medical survey of female boxing in Italy 2002–2003. Br J Sports Med 2005;39:532–6.
12. Bledsoe GH, Guohua L, Levy F. Injury risk in professional boxing. South Med J 2005;98:994–8.
13. Matser EJT, Kessels AGH, Lezak MD, et al. Acute traumatic brain injury in amateur boxing. Phys Sports Med 2000;28(1):87–92.
14. Larson LW, Melin KA, Nordstrom-Ohrberg G, et al. Acute head injuries in boxing. Acta Psychiatr Neurol Scand 1954;95(Suppl):1–42.
15. McCunney RJ, Russo PK. Brain injuries in boxers. Phys Sports Med 1984;12:53–67.
16. Critchley M. Medical aspects of boxing, particularly from a neurological standpoint. Br Med J 1957;1:357–62.
17. Sercl M, Jaros O. The mechanisms of cerebral concussion in boxing and their consequences. World Neurol 1962;3:351–7.
18. Windle WF, Groat RA. Disappearance of nerve cells after concussion. Anat Rec 1945;93:201–9.
19. Oppenheimer DR. Microscopic lesions in the brain following injury. J Neurol Neurosurg Psychiatr 1968;31:299–306.
20. Lampert PW, Hardman JM. Morphological changes in brains of boxers. JAMA 1984;251:2676–9.
21. Unterharnsheidt F. About boxing: review of historical and medical aspects. Tex Rep Biol Med 1970;28:421–95.
22. Viano DC, Casson IR, Pellman EJ, et al. Concussion in professional football: comparison with boxing head impacts – part 10. Neurosurgery 2005;57:1154–72.
23. Parkinson D. The biomechanics of concussion. Clin Neurosurg 1982;29:131–45.
24. Waliko TJ, Viano DC, Bir CA. Biomechanics of the head for Olympic boxer punches to the face.

25. Miller LP, Hayes RL. Head trauma: basic, preclinical, and clinical directions. New York: Wiley-Liss; 2001.

26. Quality Standards Subcommittee of the American Academy of Neurology. Practice parameter: the management of concussion in sports (summary statement). Neurology 1997;48:581–5.

27. Cantu RC. Guidelines for return to contact sports after a cerebral concussion. Phys Sports Med 1986;14(10):75–83.

28. McCrory P, Meeuwisse W, Johnston K, et al. Consensus statement on concussion in sport 3rd International Conference on concussion in sport held in Zurich, November 2008. Clin J Sport Med 2009;19(3):185–200.

29. Jordan BD. Increasing medical safety in boxing. In: Jordan BD, editor. Medical aspects of boxing. Boca Raton (FL): CRC Press; 1993. p. 17–21.

30. Saunders RL, Harbaugh RE. The second impact in catastrophic contact: sports head trauma. JAMA 1984;252:538–9.

31. Cantu RC, Voy R. Second impact syndrome: a risk in any sport. Phys Sports Med 1995;23:27–31.

32. Mcrory PR, Berkovic SF. Second impact syndrome. Neurology 1998;50:677–83.

33. Laurer HL, Scherbel U, Raghupathi R, et al. Second impact syndrome: myth of pathologic sequelae? J Neurotrauma 1999;16:956.

34. Martland HAS. Punch drunk. JAMA 1928;91:1103–7.

35. Roberts AH. Brain damage in boxers. London: Pitman Publishing; 1969.

36. McCrory P, Zazryn T, Cameron P. The evidence for chronic traumatic encephalopathy in boxing. Sports Med 2007;37:467–76.

37. Loosemore M, Knowles CH, Whyte GP. Amateur boxing and risk of chronic traumatic brain injury: systemic review of observational studies. Br J Sports Med 2008;42:564–7.

38. Jordan BD, Matser E, Zimmerman RD, et al. Sparring and cognitive function in professional boxers. Phys Sports Med 1996;24(5):87–98.

39. Jordan BD, Jahre C, Hauser WA. Serial computed tomography in professional boxers. J Neuroimaging 1992;2:181–5.

40. Orrison WW, Hanson EH, Alamo T, et al. Traumatic brain injury: a review and high-field MRI findings in 100 unarmed combatants using a literature-based checklist approach. J Neurotrauma 2009;26:1–13.

41. Mendez MF. The neuropsychiatric aspects of boxing. Int J Psychiatry 1995;25:249–62.

42. LaCava G. Boxer's encephalopathy. J Sports Med Phys Fitness 1963;168(3):87–92.

43. Casson IR, Siegel O, Sham R, et al. Brain damage in modern boxers. JAMA 1984;251:2663–7.

44. Casson IR, Sham R, Campbell EA, et al. Neurological and CT evaluation of knocked-out boxers. J Neurol Neurosurg Psychiatr 1982;45:170–4.

45. Sironi VA, Scotti G, Ravagnati L, et al. CT scan and EEG findings in professional pugilists: early detection of cerebral atrophy in young boxers. J Neurosurg Sci 1982;26:165–8.

46. Ross RJ, Cole M, Thompson JS, et al. Boxers – computed tomography, EEG and neurosurgical evaluation. JAMA 1983;249:211–3.

47. Jordan BD, Zimmerman RD. Computed tomography, magnetic resonance imaging comparisons in boxers. JAMA 1990;263:1670–4.

48. Zhang L, Heier LA, Zimmerman RD, et al. Diffusion anisotropy changes in the brains of professional boxers. AJNR Am J Neuroradiol 2006;27:2000–4.

49. Kemp PM, Houston AS, Macleod MA, et al. Cerebral perfusion and psychometric testing in military amateur boxers and controls. J Neurol Neurosurg Psychiatr 1995;59:368–74.

50. Jordan BD, Dane SD, Rowen AJ, et al. SPECT scanning in professional boxers. J Neuroimaging 1999;9:59–60.
51. Provenzano F, Jordan BD, Alderson P, et al. Mapping chronic traumatic brain injury in boxers: an SPM analysis of FDG PET scans. J Nucl Med 2007; 48(Suppl 2):259.
52. Vagnozzi R, Signoretti S, Tavazzi B, et al. Temporal window of metabolic brain vulnerability to concussion: a pilot 1H- magnetic resonance spectroscopy study in concussed athletes – part III. Neurosurgery 2008;62:1286–96.
53. Thomassen A, Juul-Jensen P, Olivarius B, et al. Neurological electroencephalographic and neuropsychological examination of 53 former amateur boxers. Acta Neurol Scand 1979;60:352–62.
54. Brookler KH, Itil T, Jordan BD. Electrophysiologic testing in boxers. In: Jordan BD, editor. Medical aspects of boxing. Boca Raton (FL): CRC Pres; 1993. p. 207–14.
55. Corsellis JAN, Bruton CJ, Freeman-Browne C. The aftermath of boxing. Psychol Med 1973;3:270–303.
56. Corsellis JAN. Posttraumatic dementia in Alzheimer's disease. In: Jatzman R, Terry RD, Bick K, editors. Senile dementia and related disorders. New York: Raven Press; 1978. p. 125–33.
57. Roberts GW, Allsop D, Bruton C. The occult aftermath of boxing. J Neurol Neurosurg Psychiatr 1990;53:373–8.
58. Tokuda T, Ikeda S, Yanugesa N, et al. Re-examination of ex-boxer's brain using immunohistochemistry with antibodies to amyloid beta protein and tau protein. Acta Neuropathol 1991;82:280–5.
59. Dale GE, Leigh PN, Luthert P, et al. Neurofibrillary tangles in dementia pugilistica are ubiquinated. J Neurol Neurosurg Psychiatr 1991;54:116–8.
60. Uhl GR, McKinney M, Hedreen JC, et al. Dementia pugilistic: loss of basal forebrain cholinergic neurons and cortical cholinergic markers. Ann Neurol 1982;12:99.
61. Uryu K, Chen XH, Martinez D, et al. Multiple proteins implicated in neurodegenerative diseases accumulate in axons after brain trauma in humans. Exp Neurol 2007;208:185–92.
62. Saija A, Hayes RL, Lyeth BG, et al. The effects of concussive head injury on central cholinergic neurons. Brain Res 1988;452:303–11.
63. Smith CM, Swash M. Possible biochemical basis of memory disorder in Alzheimer's disease. Neurology 1978;3:471–3.
64. Nicoll JAR, Roberts GW, Graham DI. Apolipoprotein Ee4 allele is associated with deposition of amyloid beta protein following head injury. Nat Med 1995;1:135–7.
65. Mayeaux R, Ottoman R, Maestre G, et al. Synergistic effects of traumatic head injury and apoplipoprotein e4 in patients with Alzheimer's disease. Neurology 1995;45:555–7.
66. Katzman R, Galosko DR, Saitoh T, et al. Apolipoprotein e4 and head trauma: synergistic or additive risks? Neurology 1996;46:889–92.
67. Jordan BD, Kanick AB, Horwich MS, et al. Apolipoprotein e4 and fatal cerebral amyloid angiopathy associated with dementia puglistica. Ann Neurol 1995;38: 698–9.
68. Jordan BD, Relkin NR, Ravdin LD, et al. Apolipoprotein Ee4 associated with chronic traumatic brain injury in boxing. JAMA 1997;278:136–40.
69. Jordan BD. Genetic susceptibility to brain injury in sports. A role for genetic testing in athletes. Phys Sports Med 1998;28(2):25–6.

# Nonneurologic Emergencies in Boxing

Domenic F. Coletta, Jr., MD[a,b,c]

- Boxing • Emergencies • Trauma • Cardiac • Psychiatric

Ringside medicine encompasses a wide variety of issues and historically, physicians who work boxing and mixed martial arts (MMA) events have come from all of the various specialties in medicine, from Family Practice to Neurosurgery and even Obstetrics & Gynecology. But what they all must have in common is the ability to recognize and manage not only the basic noncritical injuries and conditions in this sport, but those rare, more serious medical and traumatic emergencies that may occur in the course of a boxing match. Although most of what a ringside physician does requires as much common sense as it does a basic medical knowledge, the most important element of a ringside physician's armamentarium is his or her ability to handle what could be a life-threatening or possibly career-ending emergency.[1] Therefore, no matter what discipline of medicine a doctor who works in combative sports specializes in, experience in trauma assessment and care certainly is crucial and it is highly recommended that a ringside physician at one time or another success-fully completes courses in Advanced Cardiac and Trauma Life Support.

Unlike most sports medicine physicians, doctors in professional boxing and MMA are often scrutinized more closely by the Press, the public, and even their own medical organizations. The American Medical Association as well as other voices in and outside of medicine have at one time or another proclaimed objection to the concept of these combative sports in general and therefore, those physicians who choose to work in professional boxing and MMA must be extremely diligent in performing the task they are assigned to do, that being, protecting the health and safety of the boxer. This task can often be difficult, considering the magnitude of excitement at some of these contests, as well as the nature of the athlete, which all too often is one of fanat-ical courage and determination to win or at least remain standing until the end of the match.

Professional boxing and MMA have done an admirable job in promoting safety stan-dards in their particular sports. Through the efforts of organizations such as The

[a] New Jersey State Athletic Control Board, PO Box 180, Trenton, NJ 08675, USA
[b] American Association of Professional Ringside Physicians, 40 Heights Road, Suite 201 Darien, CT 06820, USA
[c] Cape Emergency Physicians, Department of Emergency Medicine, Cape Regional Medical Center, 2 Stone Harbor Boulevard, Cape May Court House, NJ 08210, USA
*E-mail address:* dcmd2@comcast.net

Clin Sports Med 28 (2009) 579–590
doi:10.1016/j.csm.2009.06.001                    sportsmed.theclinics.com
0278-5919/09/$ – see front matter © 2009 Elsevier Inc. All rights reserved.

Association of Boxing Commissions (ABC) and the American Association of Professional Ringside Physicians (AAPRP), guidelines have been created to help reduce injuries in such athletic events that can often have brutal activity associated with it. However, like any sport, injuries occur during the normal course of competition and, unfortunately, an occasional life-threatening emergency may arise. Although the most common medical emergencies in boxing are injuries from closed head trauma, in this article on Medical Aspects of Boxing those infrequent but potentially catastrophic nonneurologic conditions are reviewed along with some less serious "emergencies" that the physician must be prepared to address.

## THE BLEEDING BOXER

Second only to head trauma, the next most frequent injury in boxing and MMA involves bleeding from lacerations or subcutaneous blood, also known as a hematoma. Facial and scalp lacerations are dealt with in much more depth in another article of this issue. However, although a laceration may not represent a true life-threatening emergency, if that wound is located in such a place that it obstructs the vision of the fighter, it renders him or her more vulnerable to that injury which, in fact, could become an acutely dangerous medical condition. Therefore, it cannot be stressed enough that ringside physicians become adept at evaluating which cuts require stoppage of a fight and which ones do not present significant danger to the athlete who wishes to continue.

Hematomas are also not considered emergent conditions unless the collection of blood is located in an area that causes significant obstruction to the boxer's vision and places him or her at a disadvantage and thus in a dangerous situation. Unlike what might occur in a Hollywood movie scene, hematomas in boxing are not incised and drained to allow the boxer better vision. Hematomas are in fact treated with ice or compression of a cold piece of metal to help reduce the swelling. Cornermen should be instructed specifically to not rub the cold metal or ice pack against the hematoma in an attempt to flatten the swelling as this just spreads the bleeding further throughout the subcutaneous tissue.

## ORAL, OCULAR, AND EAR/NOSE/THROAT TRAUMA

This topic is dealt with in more detail in other articles of this issue; however, it is vital to discuss those life-threatening emergencies that can occur as a result of trauma to the face and neck.

Fractures involving the mandible bone are not an uncommon occurrence in boxing or MMA, and pose a potential significant danger in terms of airway obstruction and compromise to the victim of such an injury. Severe, especially bilateral mandibular fractures can create enough edema, bleeding, or relaxation of the muscles of the tongue and oral pharynx to create obstruction at the level of the upper airway in the mouth. Likewise, a fractured free-floating maxilla bone can also fall back far enough to create airway obstruction.[2] Isolated dental evulsions are at risk of being aspirated, especially by the boxer who is exhausted and breathing laborlessly, and this can also become an emergent pulmonary issue.[3] Any amount of oral-pharyngeal bleeding that is not well controlled creates the possibility of airway compromise and necessitates that a fight be discontinued. The use of a high-quality, dental-fitted mouthpiece cannot be overemphasized in light of the potential oral injuries that can occur in boxing. In fact, many experts believe that a good mouthpiece is the most important piece of protective equipment a boxer can have.

When transporting a boxer who has had a significant oral-pharyngeal injury to the Emergency Department, it is essential that he or she not be laid supine so as to avoid further possible airway obstruction. The boxer must be transported upright, often with a chin lift/jaw thrust maneuver applied to assure airway patency. If a cervical spine injury is of significant concern and the boxer **must** be placed in a supine posi- tion for transport, then it is absolutely critical that the physician or a well-trained para- medic accompanies the fighter with airway equipment, including suction, readily available. In the unlikely event of an unconscious boxer with significant facial trauma and airway compromise, oral-tracheal intubation should be attempted to establish a patent airway. A practitioner less experienced with airway management may choose to insert a laryngeal mask airway (LMA) tube rather than intubate the fighter; however, in the face of significant oral trauma this may not be the best method of choice. Retrograde intubation using a guide wire or creating a surgical airway by per- forming a cricothyrotomy may be alternative life-saving maneuvers in this type of scenario when performed by an experienced physician. A detailed description of these advanced airway techniques is beyond the scope of this article but can be found in most trauma manuals.

A nasal fracture, a common occurrence in combative sports, usually does not constitute a true emergency and is usually not reason enough to halt a fight. Severe epistaxis, however, with the potential for aspiration of blood, does fall into the same category as discussed earlier with uncontrolled oral-pharyngeal bleeding. Other urgent situations involving a broken nose include open fracture (a wound on the nose with suspected fracture underneath) and the presence of cerebral spinal fluid rhi- norrhea, which could indicate disruption of the base of the skull, a very unlikely event in a boxing match.

Direct blunt trauma to the anterior portion of the neck can be a true recipe for disaster. Although most good boxers protect their necks with their upright fists, if a punch from an opponent should land near or directly on the boxer's larynx, signifi- cant acute or delayed complications can occur. One of the most devastating injuries that could potentially occur in a combat sport is the fractured larynx, diagnosed easily by the presence of subcutaneous emphysema, hoarseness, a palpable fracture in the midline of the neck, and of course any respiratory distress on the part of the trauma victim. Emergency airway management is critical and is best accomplished in the setting of an Emergency Department or trauma center; however, if emergent intuba- tion becomes necessary at the scene of the event or in transport to the hospital due to severe respiratory distress, apnea, or impending cardiopulmonary arrest, then oral-tracheal intubation for placement of an airway should be attempted initially as it has the fewest complications.[4] If intubation attempts fail and the boxer's mental status and respiratory status continue to deteriorate, prehospital cricothyrotomy is indicated, especially if the transit time to the nearest Emergency Department is prolonged. As long as an endotracheal tube can be passed distal to the laryngeal fracture, the emer- gent situation should be manageable at that point. In the case of a blunt traumatic injury to the larynx that does not cause an obvious fracture, early intubation may still be the best option as delayed laryngeal edema or laryngeal hematomas can cause progressive airway compromise and, especially for long transport time, turn a non- urgent situation into a true respiratory emergency.

## BLUNT CHEST TRAUMA

A well-conditioned, properly trained boxer enters the ring of combat with a strong muscular cover over his or her thoracic cage and the instinctive tendency to protect the chest wall by fighting with upright arms. For these reasons, a serious injury from blunt chest trauma in a boxing match would seem extremely unlikely. In fact, pulmonary or myocardial contusion secondary to injury in a boxing ring is almost inconceivable. What may occur, however, and probably happens more than is detected by medical personnel, is that a boxer suffers a fractured rib from a hard punch that hits the thorax directly. A fractured rib, for the most part, does not constitute a medical emergency even though it can be a very painful condition that can inhibit a person's respiratory drive and eventually lead to atelectasis or pneumonia. Two scenarios, however, do exist in which a rib injury can evolve into a life-threatening complication. The first of these, rib fractures to the inferior left thoracic cage that cause a laceration to the spleen, is discussed in more depth elsewhere in this article. The other true emergency situation involving a fractured rib is that of a tension pneumothorax, one of the leading causes of death due to blunt thoracic trauma.[5] Whereas most parenchymal lung injuries from a blunt force will seal spontaneously, in the case of a tension pneumothorax air from the punctured lung enters the pleural space without a means of exit. This rapidly progressive and devastating situation manifests with certain crucial signs and symptoms the ringside physician must be aware of. A fighter experiencing a tension pneumothorax from a rib injury will commonly have significant respiratory distress due to the collapse of the affected lung. There will be decreased breath sounds on the side of the collapse as well as tracheal deviation contralaterally due to mediastinal shifts from air pressure in the thoracic cage. As the tension pneumothorax progresses, subcutaneous air can often be palpated and the person will likely show signs of shock including hypotension due to impaired venous return from a kinked inferior or superior vena cava, resulting in decreased cardiac output.[6] This presentation will also often be apparent by neck vein distension and—a late sign—cyanosis. This is a clinical diagnosis and life-saving treatment should not be delayed by waiting for transport to a facility to confirm the diagnosis radiologically. The simple procedure that must be performed to turn a boxer's condition around from potential cardiopulmonary arrest to restored respiratory comfort is the insertion of a 12- or 14-gauge angiocath needle into the second intercostal space in the midclavicular line on the side of the tension pneumothorax. This maneuver, which should be followed by an auditory rush of air and dramatic improvement in the boxer's overall condition, should then obviously be followed with immediate transportation to a trauma center for chest tube placement. There are few things in medicine and trauma that give such instant gratification on both the part of the physician and his or her patient as decompression of a tension pneumothorax and for this reason, the 12- or 14-gauge needle should be part of the equipment carried by any ringside physician.

Another potential emergency from blunt trauma in sports occurs when a direct blow strikes the peristernal area over the heart causing cardiac arrest. This catastrophic condition, known as commodio cordis, has been described in the medical literature and reported on sports pages around the world. The usual scenario for this injury, with its unfortunately devastating consequences, occurs most frequently on the baseball diamond when a batted ball strikes the pitcher in the chest. The blow to the heart, which occurs just before the T-wave repolarization during electronic conduction, results in a malignant arrhythmia, most likely ventricular defibrillation.[7] Without immediate defibrillation of the cardiac arrest victim, resuscitation is often unsuccessful. Although commodio cordis may be an unlikely occurrence in boxing and MMA arenas, it is still one more compelling argument to have emergency medical personnel and automatic external defibrillators present at all such competitions.

## BLUNT ABDOMINAL TRAUMA

In a recent pro-football game, a quarterback started to experience symptoms of light-headedness before the end of the contest, and was eventually diagnosed and treated for a splenic injury suffered at some point of time during the game when he was struck in the abdominal wall. Whereas blunt abdominal trauma is actually responsible for 10% of all trauma deaths, the vast majority have been from motor vehicle crashes followed by accidental falls and assaults.[8] Sports-related emergencies due to abdominal trauma certainly do occur, and it is not unlikely during a boxing or MMA match that a fighter will suffer a significant punch or kick to the left or right upper quadrant of the abdomen where two very vulnerable, solid organs exist; the spleen and the liver. In the case of a liver injury, which most likely would occur from an unprotected uppercut punch to the right costophrenic region or upper quadrant of the abdomen, the boxer often is unable to continue to fight due to the pain incurred as well as respiratory difficulty in most cases. The post-fight evaluation is very important, and possibly a computed tomography (CT) scan of the abdomen may be needed if the boxer remains symptomatic. In most cases, however, a hepatic contusion or small laceration to the liver can be handled conservatively without surgical intervention. A fighter cannot compete after a significant hepatic injury until he or she has been completely cleared by a general surgeon or sports medicine specialist. The spleen, on the other hand, is the most frequently damaged intraperitoneal organ, and the consequences of splenic injuries can be much more serious when the blunt trauma force is to the left upper quadrant of the abdomen. The spleen is much more likely to rupture or bleed significantly; creating a splenic hematoma and therefore, the ringside physician needs to be aware of a potential consequence of unprotected body punches to the left upper quadrant. The scenario is not likely to occur, due to the usually strong musculature of a boxer's abdominal wall as well as the instinct to protect the torso from body punches. However, because the onset of symptoms from splenic hematoma or rupture can sometimes be delayed from hours to even weeks later, physicians who treat these athletes need to keep a high index of suspicion for this injury, especially in the boxer who complains of intermittent abdominal pain, lightheadedness, or unexplained syncopal episodes. It is extremely important in pre-fight evaluations to make sure the combatant has not had a recent or current diagnosis of infectious mononucleosis, which can enlarge the spleen, or coagulopathy of any nature, which can cause profound consequences even with trivial amounts of trauma to the abdominal wall.

The classic signs of abdominal pain, hypotension, and tachycardia in splenic rupture may not be that apparent immediately after a fight in a boxer who may have an increased heart rate or distracting pain from other injuries secondary to the combative competition he or she has just completed. Knowing a boxer's pre-fight blood pressure may be helpful in determining whether the normotensive or hypotensive blood pressure readings after a fight are significant to indicate possible hemodynamic injury and potential shock. If a splenic injury is even being considered due to a witnessed abdominal trauma along with the proper symptomatology, that boxer must be sent to an Emergency Department for an evaluation, which would include a CT scan of the abdomen for a stable patient or the ultrasound FAST (Focused Assessment with Sonography in Trauma) examination for the patient whose vital signs indicate impending shock. Although the ultimate treatment for a ruptured spleen includes blood products and emergent surgery, prehospital fluids should be started when feasible. How soon to run the infusion of normal saline or lactated Ringer solution when active intraperitoneal bleeding is suspected depends on the condition of the patient and transport time to the nearest hospital. A swoop and scoop philosophy should be implemented by rescue squads and ringside physicians at the scene when significant blunt abdominal trauma has occurred and hospital transport times are reasonably short.

Due to the high tolerance of pain in most boxers and in light of the fact that there may be multiple other injuries involved (including head trauma with altered sensorium), it is extremely important that the physician's abdominal examination be a diligent one when suspecting significant traumatic injury. The most valuable physical finding in abdominal trauma comes from palpation; however, it is difficult sometimes to distinguish between abdominal wall muscular trauma and intraperitoneal injury. It can sometimes help to have the boxer contract his or her rectus muscles to determine if the tenderness is muscular or due to visceral injury. It is also important to bear in mind that as many as 20% of patients with left lower rib fractures will have splenic injury, so palpation that creates pain to the thoracic cage in that region should also create suspicion of intra-abdominal pathology. However, it must be kept in mind that the initial sign or symptom of a severe splenic injury can be a syncopal episode that occurs days or weeks later after the contest and therefore should be taken seriously in any boxer or MMA participant.

Although not nearly as vulnerable an organ to blunt trauma as the spleen, the kidney can certainly also be injured during combative sports contests. Renal contusion can occur from a direct blow to the flank of a boxer's abdomen and may also go unnoticed in a post-fight examination unless flank hematuria is reported to the physician. Grossly bloody urine requires an immediate investigation of a genitourinary system, and a perfectly clear yellow specimen on visual inspection usually indicates there is no significant renal damage. The combination of continued costovertebral angle tenderness with blood-tinged urine or microscopic hematuria should prompt the physician to order an abdominal CT examination and probably consult a urologist. Much like liver injuries, renal trauma is usually managed conservatively with observation and a ban on any physical contact until reevaluation by the particular specialist.

Finally, a brief discussion of genital injury from blunt trauma is warranted because occasionally, a boxer will receive an accidental punch or kick below the waistline. For this reason, female fighters in almost all jurisdictions are prohibited from entering the ring when pregnant. The obvious potential for injury to the gravid uterus is unacceptable in this sport. Male boxers, despite the protective equipment used in the sport, still remain vulnerable to scrotal injuries, which in most cases result in a benign hematocele; a painful, often echymotic scrotal mass secondary to accumulation of blood within the tunica vaginalis.[9] The boxer's testicles are usually not injured from minor blunt force mechanisms due to testicular mobility and the protective cremasteric reflex, as well as the encapsulation of each testicle by a fibrous cover. Trauma-induced testicular torsion, however, has been reported and therefore should be considered by a ringside physician in his or her differential diagnosis when blunt scrotal trauma has occurred in a boxing ring. Any fighter with the complaint of testicular pain after a bout should be sent immediately to a hospital where color flow duplex Doppler ultrasound can be carried out to evaluate intratesticular blood flow. Immediate urological surgery may be necessary to salvage a torsed testicle.

## ORTHOPEDIC TRAUMA

A discussion of the myriad of orthopedic injuries that can occur in combative sports is well beyond the scope of this article. Nonetheless, it is important to stress the need for the ringside physician to be able to recognize various joint, muscle, and bone injuries as, not unlike the visually impaired boxer, certain orthopedic injuries can put a fighter at a significant disadvantage and thus lead to one of the more potential emergency issues previously discussed. Therefore, any boxer with a significant orthopedic complaint either before or during a bout should not be allowed to continue in that athletic competition. As far as true emergencies are concerned in musculoskeletal trauma, certainly the dislocated joint (usually a shoulder in boxing and elbow or ankle in MMA) that has any neurovascular compromise must be reduced immediately.[10] Reduction techniques can be learned easily by the nonorthopedic ringside physician and usually performed without difficulty in the exhausted, relaxed fighter whose pain tolerance is usually quite high to begin with.[11]

Probably the only life-threatening orthopedic injury that could conceivably occur in a boxing ring is a cervical spine fracture from a direct blow to the head or neck. The studies showing that the incidence of cervical spine fracture in blunt trauma patients is between 1% and 6% have been done for the most part on victims of vehicular trauma.[12] Sports-related cervical trauma injury is more commonly seen in areas such as competitive motocross racing, downhill skiing, and other high-speed sports, and rarely as a result of an injury in a boxing ring. It is, however, important for the ringside physician to observe closely how a boxer goes to ground after a knockout punch and determine as quickly as possible once in the ring whether a mechanism for cervical spine injury is realistic or not. It would be easy to say that every fallen boxer should be placed on a long board with a cervical spine collar used to immobilize the neck, but realistically in only the very cooperative boxer or the unconscious boxer can this be achieved without difficulty. Although immediate neck in-line traction should be placed on a boxer who has been knocked down or knocked out, if their fall to the canvas did not include what would appear to have been severe head or neck trauma, and the boxer is aroused without any complaint, it is probably unnecessary to keep him or her in spinal immobilization for transport to the hospital. On the other hand, any boxer who awakens from a knockout with neck pain or any neurologic complaints in the extremities must be placed in spinal immobilization for transport to a nearby hospital with neurosurgical availability. Spinal immobilization with a long board and cervical collar is not without its own inherent complications at times. The risk of aspiration from emesis in an unconscious boxer, as well as the overall restriction of a boxer's respirations from the straps used to hold them to the board, can be quite problematic, and prehospital personnel should be diligent in only immobilizing those trauma victims that truly need to have this safety measure in transport.

Although the most serious outcomes of C-spine fractures are certainly quadriplegia and quadraparesis,[13] airway management considerations must be the priority for the physician at ringside before transportation to the Emergency Department. If an airway is not established in the unconscious apneic boxer, then the outcome from any neurosurgical intervention will not make a difference in the long-term picture. The technique of choice for establishing an airway in a boxer with a suspected cervical spine fracture is oral-tracheal intubation with direct visualization of the vocal cords while in-line traction is being applied by a second health care provider.[14] This can best be done in the setting of an Emergency Department using rapid sequence induction before intubation; however, in-field attempts are necessary if the boxer is apneic or the transport time to the hospital is prolonged. Other alternative methods include the LMA tube, retrograde intubation, or surgical cricothyrotomy in the hands of an experienced emergency care provider.

## ACUTE PSYCHOTIC EMERGENCIES

In the eyes of the general public who may not be boxing fans, the athletes who compete in combative sports such as boxing and MMA are thought to probably have some underlying mental health issues that lead them to participate in this type of activity. This notion cannot be further from the truth, as the vast majority of young men and women who box are emotionally well adjusted and intelligent individuals. However, from time to time, both in the ring and after a bout, certain psychiatric episodes are apparent and must be addressed. Whereas anxiety disorders are the most prevalent of the psychoses that plaque young adults,[15] major depression, panic disorders, and posttraumatic stress syndrome as well as bipolar disease are just as prevalent in the athletic community as in the general public. Even the casual sports fan is aware of a few instances in the recent past when a boxer elicited somewhat bizarre behavior while in the ring during a competition. The most memorable instance of an acute psychotic episode in the ring occurred during a heavyweight championship fight some years ago when one of the boxers suddenly started to elicit emotional outbursts and wandered through the ring with arms at his side in an apparent mental health crisis. Although extremely rare, this type of behavior requires immediate intervention by both the referee and the ringside physician to prevent a catastrophic injury to that emotionally and physically defenseless boxer. However, the responsibility of a good ringside physician extends beyond what happens in the ring and becomes important in both the pre- and post-bout mental health evaluations. In the pre-participation physical examination, once the physician has established a sense of trust and confidentially with the boxer, the most important question they can ask is "are you ready to compete in this boxing contest?" Any boxer who hesitates to answer this question or indicates in even the most subtle way that they are not emotionally ready to fight should not be permitted to get in the ring on that occasion. The examination after the fight also becomes an important responsibility for the physician as well as the boxer's managers and cornermen if it is determined that this boxer has potential psychiatric issues and needs some intervention. It is certainly not unusual to see a fighter have outbursts of anger or periods of serious depression with crying episodes after losing a big contest. These signs certainly do not necessarily indicate that an acute psychosis has occurred; however, continued symptoms of uncontrollable anger, concentration disturbances, loss of appetite, loss of interest or lack of pleasure from the sport, insomnia, and other recurrent emotional red flags should give a boxer's physician or manager reason to be concerned about a potential psychiatric problem.[16] Other situations that require diligent observation to rule out a potential suicidal ideation include the posttraumatic stress disorder that can be seen often in a boxer whose opponent has died in the ring as a result of their combat, and the postconcussion depression that occurs from multiple head traumas. Also, the boxer whose career ends with a devastating loss or severe injury can be known to fall into a deep depression and may require mental health counseling. In any case, it is important for physicians in ringside medicine to be aware of some of the symptoms associated with suicide including feelings of hopelessness, severe anxiety and panic attacks, impaired concentration, psychomotor agitation or depression, insomnia, and a general disconnection with friends and family.[17] Because the pre- and post-fight, physical examinations may be the only time a boxer gets to see a physician, it is essential for those physicians in ringside medicine to be as complete as possible in their evaluations both from a physical and mental health standpoint.

## CARDIAC EMERGENCIES

Any discussion of medical emergencies in sports should include the topic of life-threatening cardiac events that can cause death or severe disability in an athlete during competition. Sudden cardiac death, defined as an unexpected death due to cardiac causes that occurs rapidly in a person with known or unknown heart disease in whom no previously diagnosed fatal condition is apparent,[18] seems to be most often reported at the level of high school, college, and amateur sports. Although it is not a likely scenario in the professional ranks of boxing, due to the fact that most of these athletes have been competing for several years before reaching the professional level, the discussion of sudden cardiac death is nonetheless important as it regards to this article, and knowledge of how to manage a victim in cardiopulmonary arrest is crucial for any physician working a sporting event. Professional fighters are among the very best conditioned athletes in sports and in nearly all cases have spent numerous hours in the gym as well as several rounds in an amateur ring. Therefore, it is more likely that a spectator at a boxing match will have a cardiac arrest than will one of the athletes who are competing. However, whether it is a person from the crowd whom the physician feels ethically responsible to assist, or the boxer who suddenly collapses in a ring and has no pulse or respiration, it is the quick response of ringside medical personnel that can make the difference.

The most common electrophysiological mechanism that leads to sudden cardiac death is the malignant arrhythmias of ventricular fibrillation or pulseless ventricular tachycardia. In the case of young, seemingly healthy athletes, most cases of sudden cardiac death are due to either structural abnormalities of the heart, most likely hypertrophic cardiomyopathy (HCM) or, less commonly, the inherited arrhythmia conditions such as long QT syndrome and Brugada syndrome. HCM, an autosomal dominant genetic disorder, is the single greatest cause of sudden cardiac death in young, previously asymptomatic athletes and therefore should be screened for during the physical examination of any boxer. At present, most state and tribal boxing commissions require an electrocardiogram (EKG) as a baseline test before a boxer gets his or her professional license. However, the EKG is not an accurate screening modality for this disease. Any boxer who has a heart murmur on auscultation of the chest certainly should be considered for a further workup with a 2D echocardiogram to rule out HCM. The mechanism of sudden cardiac death in HCM is not entirely understood, but it is thought that somehow the hypertrophy of the walls of the heart chambers may provide the substrate for the lethal arrhythmia that occurs. Probably the most efficient screening tool a physician has for this life-threatening disease is the history given by the athlete. Any boxer with a history of recurrent syncopal episodes, a family history of sudden cardiac death, documented palpitations or murmurs, or evidence of ventricular ectopy on stress testing should be worked up further for HCM.

Long QT syndrome and Brugada syndrome are conditions in which the athletes have no apparent structural heart disease but have a primary electrophysiological abnormality predisposing them to a lethal arrhythmia, usually ventricular fibrillation. The clinical course in Long QT syndrome can be variable with some patients remaining asymptomatic throughout their lives, yet others experiencing syncopal episodes related to torsade de pointes, a form of ventricular arrhythmia, and sudden death. Because vigorous physical activity has been associated with an increased risk in sudden cardiac deaths in patients with long QT syndrome,[18] it becomes important that the physician receive a detailed history from the boxer of any previous syncopal episodes or a family history of sudden cardiac death. That history coupled with the EKG criteria for diagnosis of this malady should certainly prompt the physician to have a full evaluation of that boxer by a cardiologist before any athletic competition.

Brugada syndrome, which is most commonly seen in young, otherwise healthy men often of Asian decent, is another disorder characterized by sudden cardiac death, and can be associated with one of several EKG patterns characterized by an incomplete right bundle branch block and ST elevations in the anterior pericardial leads.[19]

Screening for this rare but deadly syndrome should also include a complete history and knowledge of such EKG abnormalities.

Because screening for these unusual cardiac anomalies is difficult to say the least and possibly impractical for every athlete who competes, the next best solution is for medical personnel at such events to be qualified and prepared in resuscitation techniques. Without question, the most important element of successful resuscitation in the victim of sudden cardiac death is the availability of an automatic external defibrillator. It is also advisable that all physicians who practice sports medicine be proficient in the fundamentals of emergency health care (ABCs: airway, breathing, circulation). Establishing an airway in the unconscious or apneic athlete is always a priority. From the simple chin lift/jaw thrust maneuver, to insertion of an LMA tube, to the more advanced techniques of endotracheal intubation and cricothyrotomy, the ringside physician **must** feel comfortable with the overall concept of airway management. Once a patent airway has been created, the next step is to ventilate and oxygenate a fallen victim. Oxygen at ringside has been stressed throughout the years in light of the presumed advantage it gives to the unconscious boxer who has had cerebral injury and often may exhibit brief seizure activity after a knockout. The final component of the ABCs, which is circulation, entails the initial use of chest compressions and hemorrhage control immediately followed, if necessary, by the institution of intravenous fluids, antiarrhythmic medication and, most importantly, defibrillation as indicated. Although not every ringside physician will be an expert in the art of resuscitation of a victim of cardiac arrest, all doctors who work in these venues should at least feel comfortable with knowing the basic information required to treat such emergencies.

**EMERGENCY PREPAREDNESS**

Through the years, the AAPRP has made multiple recommendations to help improve safety standards in the sport of professional boxing. Among these recommendations have been the necessity of minimum medical requirements, the suggestion of using oversized gloves during sparring, and comments on how much body weight gain or loss before a fight is acceptable. However, among the most important requirements that the AAPRP has recommended and that most state and tribal boxing commissions have always adhered to is to have the presence of an ambulance with paramedics at all times in every venue where professional boxing or MMA bouts are held. In those jurisdictions where skilled paramedics are available at these contests the ringside physician can often step back and take more of a supervisory role, allowing a good paramedic team to manage the situation. In fact it is very important that a physician, depending on his or her level of expertise in emergency management, knows when to take over the hands on aspect at a scene and when to back off and not be obstructive to prehospital providers. In venues that provide emergency medical technicians (EMTs) as their rescue squad workers instead of paramedics, a physician may have to get more involved in the management of a true emergency condition. In fact, a ringside physician should strongly consider accompanying the boxer who is in extremis to the Emergency Department when being transported by EMTs rather than paramedics. In either case, no boxing or MMA show should begin, or be allowed to continue without the ambulance and rescue squad on the premises. Likewise it is advisable to hold these combative matches as near to a Level I or Level II trauma center as possible, for the health and safety of the participants. Ringside physicians should routinely know the location of the nearest Emergency Department with neurosurgical capabilities and, along with the rescue squads on the scene, know which is the best and safest way to get a boxer out of the ring, through the venue, and to the hospital. These situations should be worked out before the start of any contest and, when feasible, on-call trauma personnel at the local hospital should be given a call alerting them of the upcoming event or of an emergency that is in transit to their facility.[20] Ringside physicians should take whatever steps are necessary to ensure efficient preparedness for any and all possible emergencies that can occur at these events. From having the proper equipment available, including the 14-gauge needle to treat the rare tension pneumothorax or the tank of oxygen for the unconscious boxer who needs to save some brain cells, to convening with security and rescue personnel at the venue that may or may not be familiar, all safety precautions can only be a benefit if an emergency situation arises.

## SUMMARY

Physician presence and participation at amateur and professional boxing matches has always been a mainstay in the sport. However, over the last several years the practice of ringside medicine has taken on an even more crucial role and, in a sense, evolved into a new specialty area with its own unique practice guidelines, academic issues, and standards of care. Whereas it was always important to diagnose both the obvious as well as the more subtle, noncritical abnormalities in a pre-fight physical or during a bout, it has now become absolutely essential for the ringside physician to be able to recognize and manage true life-threatening emergencies. Fortunately, the vast majority of boxing and MMA contests do not end tragically and, in the very few that do, the death of a fighter usually occurs hours, days, or even weeks later in a hospital intensive care unit setting. Nonetheless, all ringside health professionals should be proficient in the ABCs of emergency medicine and well prepared at all times for any potentially catastrophic medical scenario that may happen.

## ACKNOWLEDGMENTS

Deepest appreciation is extended to Betty Veach for her transcription services.

## REFERENCES

1. Colpitts R.W, Goodman SJ, et al. Medical analysis—Chapter 2. In: Ringside physicians certification manual, Revised Edition. Colorado Springs (CO): United States Amateur Boxing, Inc.; 2003. p. 35–107
2. Stewart C. Maxillofacial trauma: challenges in ED diagnosis and management. Emerg Med Pract 2008;10(2):1–18.
3. Benko K. Acute dental emergencies in emergency medicine. Emerg Med Pract 2003;5(5):1–22.
4. Schaider J, Bailitz J. Neck trauma: don't put your neck on the line. Emerg Med Pract 2003;5(7):1–23.
5. American College of Surgeons. Advanced trauma life support for doctors. 7th edition. Chicago: American College of Surgeons; 2004. p. 103–29.
6. Powell MA, McMahon D, Peitzman AB. Thoracic injury. In: Peitzman AB, et al, editors. The trauma manual. Philadelphia: Lippincott-Raven Publishers; 1998. p. 199–225.
7. Perrow AD. Commodio cordis. Am J Emerg Med 2001;19(5):406–9.
8. Marx J. Blunt abdominal trauma: priorities, procedures and pragmatic thinking. Emerg Med Pract 2001;3(5):1–22.

9. Davis J, Schmeider R. An evidenced-based approach to male urogenital emergencies. Emerg Med Pract 2009;11(2):1–18.
10. Freeman L, Corley A. Orthopedic sports injuries: off the sidelines and into the emergency department. Emerg Med Pract 2003;5(4):1–21.
11. Daya M, Nakamura Y. Shoulder girdle fractures and dislocations. Emerg Med Pract 2007;9(10):1–23.
12. Beattie LK, Choi J. Acute spinal injuries: assessment and management. Emerg Med Pract 2006;8(5):1–21.
13. Snider RK, editor. Essentials of musculoskeletal care. 1st edition. Rosemont (IL): American Academy of Orthopedic Surgeons; 1997. p. 509–46.
14. Gibbs MA, Jones AE. Cervical spine injury: a state of the art approach to assessment and management. Emerg Med Pract 2001;3(10):1–19.
15. Fricchione G. Generalized anxiety disorder. N Engl J Med 2004;351:675–82.
16. Kamm RL. Interviewing principles for the psychiatrically aware sports medicine physician. Clin Sports Med 2005;24:745–66.
17. Russinoff I, Clark M. Suicidal patients: assessing and managing patients presenting with suicidal attempts or ideations. Emerg Med Pract 2004;6(8):1–17.
18. Sovari AA, Kocheril AG, McCullough PA. Sudden cardiac death. e-Medicine Cardiology article 151907. 2006;1–9.
19. Dizon JM, Saluja D, Abriel H. Brugada syndrome. e-Medicine Cardiology article 163751 2009;1–3.
20. Voy R. Medical responsibilities of the ringside physician, Chapter 1, In: Ringside physician certification manual. Revised Edition. Colorado Springs (CO): United States Amateur Boxing Inc.; 2003. p. 9–22.

# Eye Trauma in Boxing

Gustavo Corrales, MD[a],*, Anthony Curreri, MD[b]

**KEYWORDS**

- Ocular • Trauma • Coup • Contrecoup
- Retinal detachment • Refractive surgery • Boxing

## INCIDENCE AND MORBIDITY

Due to a lack of a centralized, or even local databases to record the actual incidence, nature, and outcome of eye injuries in boxing, it is difficult to quantify the impact they exert on the visual system. Ringside physicians are aware of the high incidence of acute ocular and periocular injuries with which boxers are afflicted. The most obvious and evident injuries consist of periorbital equimoses and eyelid lacerations that usually resolve with minor scarring and no visual consequences. Vision-threatening injuries, like retinal tears, require a more detailed ophthalmic examination and may be more difficult to diagnose. Many boxing injuries are monocular, and therefore may go unnoticed or be intentionally hidden by the boxer due to fear of disqualification from the sport, making the detection of these injuries more challenging.

In boxing, along with a few other sports, trauma is inherent to the nature of the sport, and therefore is considered a high-risk sport for ocular injuries.[1] It is not surprising, then, that the incidence of ocular trauma is high among boxers. Signs of ocular trauma can be found in about 66% to 76% of asymptomatic boxers, and about 21% to 58% of boxers have pronounced and vision-threatening ocular injuries.[2,3] This situation means that more than half of asymptomatic boxers have eye injuries, and a high number of them have injuries that put them at risk of permanent vision loss, such as retinal tears, retinal detachments, macular lesions, cataracts, angle injuries, and even ruptured globes (**Table 1**).[4]

The long-term morbidity of boxing ocular injuries is hard to estimate due to the lack of structured long-term follow-up of these athletes. Complications of blunt ocular trauma may develop years after the athlete has retired from the ring and no longer considered to be at risk for boxing-related injuries. For example, posttraumatic glaucoma, due to blunt trauma to the angle structures, is often insidious and may manifest many years later.

---

[a] Department of Cornea and Refractive Surgery, New York Eye and Ear Infirmary, 310 East 14th Street, New York, NY 10003, USA
[b] Ophthalmology Department, New York Eye and Ear Infirmary, 310 East 14th Street, New York, NY 10003, USA
* Corresponding author. Ophthalmology Department, New York Eye and Ear Infirmary, 310 East 14th Street, New York, NY 10003, USA
E-mail address: guscor@gmail.com (G. Corrales).

Clin Sports Med 28 (2009) 591–607
doi:10.1016/j.csm.2009.07.004
0278-5919/08/$ – see front matter © 2009 Elsevier Inc. All rights reserved.

## ANATOMIC CONSIDERATIONS AND PHYSICS

The eye sits within a pear-shaped bony orbit of about 30 mL volume. On average the orbital entrance is about 35 mm in height and 45 mm in width. The depth of the orbit ranges from 40 to 45 mm. Racial variations exist in all these measurements.[5]

The orbital bones absorb some of the total energy delivered by a blow with a blunt object that is larger than the bony orbital opening, such as a boxing glove, therefore sparing the eye of some of the impact energy. For this reason objects that are larger than the bony orbital opening were wrongly considered to be of low risk for a direct eye injury. High-speed photography has now revealed that impacting objects larger than the orbital entrance opening (ie, radius of curvature greater than 5 mm [2 in]), like a soccer ball or a boxing glove, undergo significant deformation on impact, allowing a small protuberance to enter the orbital cavity and impacting the eye globe.[6] Furthermore, a secondary suction effect created during the exiting of the protuberance from the orbital cavity causes additional stress and tearing to the intraocular structures **Fig. 1**.[7]

The eye globe is considered to be most vulnerable in its inferotemporal aspect for two reasons. First, it is the most exposed area of the eye globe because it remains relatively unprotected by the bony orbit.[8] Second, the doll's eye reflex (Bell phenomenon), which involves closing the eyelids and rolling up the eyes, leaves the inferior and temporal area of the eye exposed to a direct blow from the front or the temporal side.[9]

## MECHANISMS OF INJURY

Three different mechanisms of injury have been traditionally used to explain the injuries seen in blunt ocular trauma, although most likely all three contribute to cause ocular injury.

### Coup

Coup injury is caused by a direct blunt blow to the eye. The structures affected are basically in direct contact with the object delivering the blow. Direct blow to the external structures causes lid lacerations, corneal abrasions, conjunctival laceration, and other external injuries.

### Contrecoup

Contrecoup is a well-known mechanism of traumatic brain injury occurring away from the area of impact. A blunt injury to the skull initiates a shock wave that traverses in a straight line following the vector of impact through the intracranial tissues. Tissue damage is found at tissue interfaces. Due to anatomic similarities between the brain

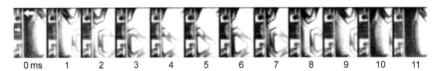

**Fig.1.** Soccer ball impact onto artificial orbit. The orbit (anterior plane, *small arrow*) is penetrated 8.1 mm by the 18 m/s (40 mph) size 3 soccer ball, which compresses on the steel plate surrounding the orbital fixture (*large arrow*). The compression phase of the ball, that drives a small knuckle of the ball into the orbit (1–4 ms), is easily seen by studying the dark triangles on the ball. During rebound, the slow orbital exit of the ball compared with the rebound from the plate (5–10 ms) produces a secondary suction effect on the orbital contents. (*From* Vinger PF, Capao Filipe JA. The mechanism and prevention of soccer eye injuries. Br J Ophthalmol 2004;88(2):167–8; with permission.)

and the eye, this mechanism of injury is also used to explain how eye injuries occur away from the area of impact. Examples of lesions caused by contrecoup include macular holes, posterior subcapsular cataracts, and macular pathology.[10] A classic injury caused by contrecoup is a superonasal retinal dialysis. This type of lesion is almost always associated with blunt ocular trauma, and is believed to be caused by a blow to the inferotemporal aspect of the globe.[8,11]

### Equatorial Expansion

According to this theory direct anteroposterior blunt trauma causes expansion of the equatorial region, where the vitreous is firmly attached to the retina at the vitreous base. Vitreous avulsion from its base is considered a pathognomonic finding of blunt ocular trauma.[12] As the equatorial sclera expands the vitreous is violently detached at its base, which may result in retinal tears, detachment of the ciliary epithelium, and retinal dialysis. Myopic eyes, which have a longer axial length and tend to have retinal conditions that predispose to retinal tears, may be more prone to develop equatorial lesions.[13]

### Eye Rupture

The rupture of an eye is a function of the peak force and the force onset rate at which a blunt object delivers its energy to the eye. A higher peak force and a faster force onset rate are directly related to the risk of eye rupture. Even though a softer object delivers more energy and intrudes deeper into the orbit, a harder object delivers the energy more rapidly, with a higher peak force and faster force onset rate, and consequently is more likely to cause significant eye injury. Experiments with baseballs help illustrate this principle (**Figs. 2** and **3**).[14] The force onset rate required to produce clinical contusion to the eye is about 750 N/ms.[15] Direct measurement of punch force in 6 professional boxing matches showed that the mean punch force ranged from 866.6 N in the Super Middleweight category to 1149.2 N in the Light Middleweight category. The boxer's weight surprisingly was not correlated to the mean punch force delivered, supporting the notion that punch velocity and technique may play an important role in determining punch force.[16] The maximal punch force was 5358 N, as delivered by a cruiserweight fighter. Therefore, ocular injuries can occur in any category of fight and a high suspicion should be maintained.

### INJURIES
### Cornea and Conjunctiva

#### Corneal abrasion
Corneal abrasion is the traumatic removal of corneal epithelial cells, and is probably a frequent corneal injury in boxing that goes undiagnosed due to its low morbidity. Depending on the size of the abrasion, it usually heals within 24 to 72 hours and does not leave a scar unless the stroma is affected. Fluorescein staining of the corneal abrasion is diagnostic and is also useful to follow its improvement. Treatment consists of ointments with or without antibiotics. While the cornea remains denuded of its epithelium, it is at risk of infections due to bacteria, fungi, and viruses. An infected corneal abrasion is called a corneal ulcer, which is sight-threatening if not treated promptly with topical antibiotics and surgery if needed. A corneal infection may penetrate into the eye causing an endophthalmitis, which may lead to irreversible blindness and even loss of the eye. A corneal abrasion may predispose the eye to recurrent corneal abrasions in the same location due to "loose" reattachment of the epithelium to the underlying basement membrane. The loose epithelium sloughs off easily with minor trauma or without any obvious cause. Recurrent corneal abrasions may cause sudden, unpredictable blurred vision and eye pain

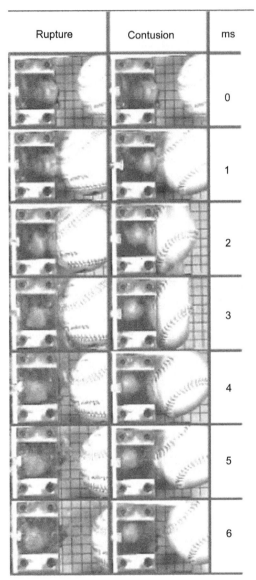

| Rupture | Contusion | ms |
|---------|-----------|-----|
| | | 0 |
| | | 1 |
| | | 2 |
| | | 3 |
| | | 4 |
| | | 5 |
| | | 6 |

**Fig. 2.** Rupture and contusion related to time in milliseconds and force onset rate.[40] (*From* Vinger PF. The mechanisms and prevention of sports eye injuries. URL: http://www.lexeye.com/pdf/Section1.pdf; with permission.)

that may interfere with a boxer's performance. Conservative treatment consists of eye ointments and artificial tears, but definitive treatment may require microstromal puncture or phototherapeutic keratectomy.[17]

### Subconjunctival hemorrhage

Subconjunctival hemorrhage occurs when a conjunctival blood vessel is disrupted, allowing intravascular blood to reach the subconjunctival space. It is of no visual

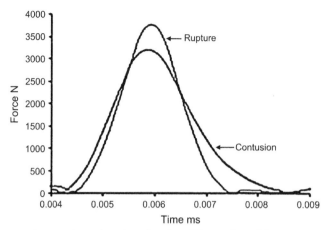

**Fig. 3.** Rupture and contusion related to time in milliseconds and force onset rate.[40] (*From* Vinger PF. The mechanisms and prevention of sports eye injuries. URL: http://www.lexeye. com/pdf/Section1.pdf; with permission.)

consequence but may be a sign of trauma to the eye, and other injuries should be sought. A subconjunctival hemorrhage resolves without intervention as the blood is reabsorbed.

### Iris and Angle Structures

#### Traumatic iritis

Traumatic iritis occurs within 24 hours after a minor to moderate blunt injury to the iris or ciliary body. Traumatic iritis is suspected by the presence of photophobia, blurred vision, and eye pain, and confirmed by the presence of anterior chamber cells and flare on slit-lamp examination. Traumatic iritis may be difficult to distinguish from a microhyphema, and both can coexist, in which case treatment of the hyphema takes precedence. Treatment consists of cycloplegics, topical steroids, and intraocular pressure lowering medications if necessary.

#### Hyphema

Trauma to the highly vascularized iris and the angle structures may lead to bleeding inside the anterior chamber. There are three clinical types of hyphema: Microhyphema can only be detected by slit-lamp examination. Microscopic red blood cells are seen floating in the anterior chamber. Macrohyphema occurs when layered red blood cells can be seen lying in the dependent area of the anterior chamber, most often the inferior angle, where blood settles by gravity. Macrohyphema may be suspected at the ringside with the help of a penlight. Final diagnosis rests on proper identification with a slit-lamp (**Fig. 4**). A total hyphema or eight-ball hyphema occurs when the whole anterior chamber is filled with blood.

The most common consequence of any hyphema is acute elevation of the intraocular pressure, which is directly related to the amount of blood in the anterior chamber. Red blood cells, fibrin, and cellular debris seem to be responsible for the obstruction of the trabecular meshwork that leads to acute ocular hypertension.[18]

Rebleeding may occur in up to 38% of cases, and usually occurs within 7 days of the initial bleed. Rebleeding is suspected by an increase in the size of the hyphema, and is associated with a poorer visual prognosis. Gonioscopy, retinal examination with scleral depression, and manipulation of the eye should be delayed for at least several

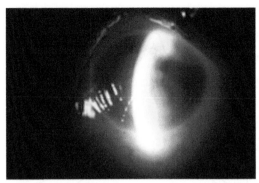

**Fig. 4.** Macrohyphema. (*From* Walton W, Von Hagen S, Grigorian R, Zarbin M. Management of traumatic hyphema. Surv Ophthalmol 2002;47(4):297–334; with permission.)

weeks to minimize the risk of a rebleed. Ultrasonography, taking care not to exert pressure on the globe, may be used to examine the posterior segment in these cases and in cases in which media opacity precludes a direct examination.

Persons with sickle cell disease or other hemoglobinopathy are at increased risk of having a rebleed. Studies have also shown that sickle cell hemoglobinopaths tend to develop higher intraocular pressures and are also more susceptible to optic nerve damage. Antifibrinolytic agents, such as aminocaproic acid and tranexamic acid, have been successfully used to prevent rebleeds in susceptible patients.[19]

Corneal blood staining occurs in the setting of hyphema with consistent elevated intraocular pressure and corneal endothelial dysfunction. This condition often takes several months to years to clear, and a corneal transplant may be indicated for visual rehabilitation.[18] Irreversible optic nerve damage with atrophy has been reported in the setting of hyphema with or without documented elevated intraocular pressure.[19]

Surgical evacuation of the hyphema is indicated in cases in which the intraocular pressure cannot be controlled with topical and oral medications, and may be sight-saving. Medical management consists of oral and topical steroids, aqueous suppressants, eye shield (not a patch), and mandatory rest.

### Angle recession, cyclodialysis, and iridodialysis

Three types of anatomic damage due to blunt trauma are detected in the anterior segment angle with the help of a gonioscopy lens. Cyclodialysis refers to a separation of the ciliary body from the scleral spur; it may lead to ocular hypotension by creating a direct path from the anterior chamber to the suprachoroidal space. Cyclodialysis can only be detected by gonioscopy and ultrasound biomicroscopy.

Angle recession is a separation between the circular and the longitudinal fibers of the ciliary body, and is associated with an increased the risk of developing chronic glaucoma. Angle recession can only be detected by gonioscopy and ultrasound biomicroscopy.

Iridodialysis refers to a tear at the iris root. Small defects may be left alone and observed. Larger defects that are aesthetically significant and cause visual problems, like glare and halos, may require surgical repair (**Fig. 5**).

Chronic glaucoma associated with traumatic angle recession occurs in about 10% of patients. Elevated intraocular pressure after blunt trauma to the angle structures may occur in two phases. The first occurs within the first year after the trauma and may be difficult to control, but often resolves on its own. The second phase occurs

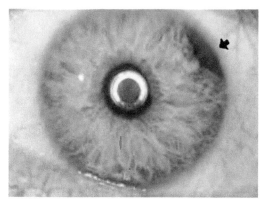

**Fig. 5.** Traumatic iridodialysis (*arrow*). (*Courtesy of* R. Ahuja, MD/Creative Commons.)

years after the trauma, and the magnitude of the elevated intraocular pressure is directly correlated with the degrees of angle recession.[20] Glaucoma onset may be insidious and occur more than 10 years after trauma. Eyes with 180° or more of traumatic angle recession are at increased risk of developing glaucoma.

There may also be an underlying genetic predisposition because in nonboxers with unilateral traumatic angle recession, up to 50% of fellow eyes develop increased intraocular pressure. Although angle recession by itself would not lead to glaucoma, it is a measure of the intensity of the injury to the adjacent trabecular meshwork, which is responsible for the outflow of the aqueous humor.[21] It is recommended that patients with traumatic angle injuries be followed annually for their lifetime.[22]

## Lens

The crystalline lens is a clear structure whose function is to focus the incoming light onto the retina. The lens has the ability to increase its power (accommodation) when nearby targets are presented to keep the image in focus on the retina.

### Cataracts

Cataracts refer to the development of opacities—sclerosis and yellowing—of the lens, and are usually an age-related change. Secondary causes of cataracts include trauma and use of steroids. Cataracts become symptomatic when they cause blurred vision, dimming of the light, glare, and halos. In general the more posterior the cataract (eg, the closer it is to the focal point of the eye), the earlier it becomes visually significant.

The most common type of traumatic cataract in boxers is the posterior subcapsular cataract (**Fig. 6**). This type accounts for 60% to 100% of all cataracts seen in boxers.[2,3] Frequently an axial stellate or rosette-shaped opacification is seen after blunt trauma (**Fig. 7**). This rosette cataract may remain stable or progress to affect the entire lens. This cataract is the most symptomatic of all, and often involves the posterior capsule making cataract surgery more challenging and increasing the chances of complications.

Other types of cataract that occur less frequently in boxers include anterior subcapsular cataract, which consists of an opacity in the anterior aspect of the lens, many times also involving the anterior capsule. Nuclear sclerosis, the most frequent type

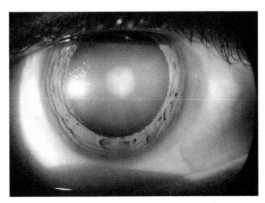

**Fig. 6.** Posterior subcapsular cataract. (*Courtesy of* R. Ahuja, MD/Creative Commons.)

of age-related cataract, can occur in young boxers.[3,23] **Table 2** shows the incidence of cataracts found in boxers in several studies.

A Vossius ring is a circular staining of the anterior capsule by pigment from the pupillary ruff that occurs when blunt trauma causes compression of the iris against the anterior capsule. This compression causes liberation and dispersion of iris pigment, which is imprinted on the anterior capsule. Vossius ring is off the visual axis and causes no visual disturbance, but remains as a telltale sign of past trauma.

### Zonular trauma
The lens is suspended within the spherical eye by a mechanism of elastic cords extending from its equator to the wall of the eye. These cords, called zonules, may be damaged during sudden equatorial expansion of the globe due to blunt trauma, causing significant stretching and even their rupture.

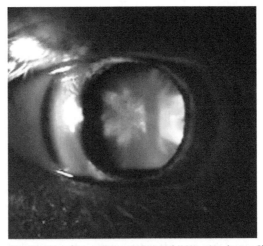

**Fig. 7.** Traumatic rosette cataract. (*From* Casser L, Perotti J. New Horizons: Slit Lamp Evaluation of the Crystalline Lens after Pupillary Dilation. http://www.opt.indiana.edu/NewHorizons. Title.html, 1997; with permission.)

| Table 1 | |
|---|---|
| **Incidence of vision-threatening ocular injuries** | |
| **Study** | **Incidence (%)** |
| Giovinazzo et al[3] | 58 |
| Smith[24] | 21 |

A sectoral zonular compromise may lead to subluxation of the lens, whereas complete zonular disruption manifests as complete dislocation of the lens into the vitreous cavity or the anterior chamber. Patients may complain of monocular diplopia and vision loss. Bianco and colleagues[23] reported a 7.3% incidence of traumatic lens dislocations in 956 Italian boxers. Zonular disruption increases the complication rate during or after cataract surgery.

### Peripheral Retina and Vitreous

Some of the most frequent and sight-threatening injuries reported in boxers are retinal detachment and retinal dialysis. A study from Wills Eye Hospital documented nine boxers, of whom eight had retinal detachments caused by blunt trauma and one a traumatic retinal tear that had not evolved into a retinal detachment.[9] One of these boxers, in whom a retinal dialysis was found, had no symptoms. Another patient with retinal detachment had a traumatic retinal dialysis in the fellow eye. These two cases underscore the fact that the absence of symptoms should not preclude the physician from performing a bilateral dilated examination routinely in these patients.

Certain retinal lesions that predispose to retinal detachments have been found more frequently in boxers than in the general population. The incidence of eyes with peripheral retinal tears was 24% in a study by Giovinazzo and colleagues[3] compared with 0% in controls. Smith found retinal holes and tears in 11% of 118 boxers.[24] In contrast, Bianco and colleagues[23] found only 6 eyes with retinal disinsertion in 956 boxers, but found none in controls. Boxers with multiple retinal tears in the same eye have been found in some studies.[3,24] Retinal tears may be caused by vitreous avulsion from its retinal attachment due to equatorial expansion by blunt trauma. Bilateral retinal detachments similarly were found in 2 of 74 (2%) boxers by Giovinazzo and colleagues,[3] and in 7 of 1912 eyes (0.36%) by Bianco and colleagues,[23] whereas none were reported by Smith (**Table 3**).[24]

Even though the incidence of retinal detachments may vary among studies, they unquestionably carry significant morbidity for the boxer. The retinal detachment of Sugar Ray Leonard brought media and public attention to this condition.[25] Maguire and Benson reported a series of 10 eyes in 9 patients with vision-threatening retinal findings who underwent retinal surgery. The final visual acuity in the affected eyes

| Table 2 | | | | |
|---|---|---|---|---|
| **Reported incidence of cataracts and lens dislocation** | | | | |
| **Study** | **n** | **Cataract (%)** | **Dislocation** | **Bilateral Involvement (%)** |
| Giovinazzo et al[3] | 74 | 20 | 0 | Not mentioned |
| Smith[24] | 68 | 10 | 0 | 5 |
| Bianco et al[23] | 956 | 3% of eyes | 7.3% of eyes | Not mentioned |
| Wedrich et al[2] | 25 | 16% | 0 | 12% of boxers |

**Table 3**
**Peripheral retinal injuries**

| Study | n | Retinal Tears (%) | Retinal Detachment (%) | Lattice Degeneration | Bilateral Findings (%) |
|---|---|---|---|---|---|
| Giovinazzo et al[3] | 74 | 24 | 2 | 3 | Not mentioned |
| Smith[24] | 68 | 11 | 0 | 1 | 1 |
| Bianco et al[23,a] | 956 | 0.06 | 0.3 | 1.3 | Not mentioned |
| Wedrich et al[2] | 25 | 24 | 0 | 0 | 20 |
| Maguire and Benson[9] | 9 | 22 | 88 | 0 | 11 |

[a] Percentage of eyes. All other numbers express percentage of boxers.

of these patients were legal for driving in 5 of the 10 boxers (20/40 or better). Three boxers had vision 20/70 to 20/400, and 2 could only see hand motion (2/10).

### Macula

The macula is responsible for the central visual acuity and has the highest density of color-sensing cells, the cones. Therefore it has a very important role in visual function. The macula may be primarily affected by a contrecoup injury or it may be secondarily affected by a peripheral retinal detachment that extends onto the visual axis.

Macular abnormalities were reported in 8% of 74 boxers by Giovinazzo and colleagues, pathologic pigmentary changes being the most frequent in 4%. Other pathologic changes found were macular cysts in 3% and macular holes in 1%.[3]

### Optic Nerve and Visual Field Defects

Visual field defects with a normal eye examination denote damage to the optic pathway within the brain and not within the eye. Field defects that respect an imaginary central vertical line are usually caused by intracranial processes, whereas those that respect an imaginary central horizontal line are usually caused by intraocular pathology, like glaucomatous optic neuropathy. Reported intracranial injuries with field defects in boxers include a left homonymous hemianopia due to a right lateral geniculate hemorrhage[26] and a right homonymous quadrantonopsia.[23]

Gross field defects may be detected ringside with a fast and simple confrontation field test. To perform this test the examiner sits or stands 1 m in front of the boxer, with the eyes at the same level. The boxer should cover the nonexamined eye and fixate on the examiner's nose with the test eye. To identify central and altitudinal (horizontal defects), the examiner asks if the entire face is visible or if some portions are missing. Then the examiner presents a target of one, two, or five fingers in each of the four quadrants and asks the patient to identify how many fingers are shown. By presenting two sets of fingers in opposing quadrants and asking the boxer the total sum of the fingers, the physician can identify extinction due to parietal lesions and subtle field defects.[27]

#### Traumatic optic neuropathy

The mechanism of traumatic optic neuropathy may be classified as direct and indirect. In the former an obvious cause for the neuropathy can be found, for example, fracture of the optic nerve canal with a bone fragment compressing the optic nerve. In the latter, there is no obvious and persistent compression of the optic nerve. Indirect optic neuropathy is most commonly caused by bony transmission of the force delivered by a blow to the brow or the superior orbital rim that extends to the optic nerve canal, with resultant trauma to the optic nerve.[28] A range of traumas have been associated with optic neuropathy, ranging from motor vehicle and bicycle accidents to fainting and assaults.[29] In many instances the trauma may be rated as mild. The hallmark triad of acute traumatic optic neuropathy consists of vision loss, an afferent pupillary defect, and optic nerve edema after trauma. The vision may improve in mild cases, but severe cases usually do not recover useful vision in the affected eye. The optic nerve head progresses to pallor over the course of 6 to 8 weeks, making its detection and diagnosis difficult. Optic nerve edema was found in 6.6% of eyes of 920 Italian boxers by Bianco and colleagues.[23] These findings are most likely to be related to indirect traumatic optic neuropathy in these healthy athletes. Improved reporting would be necessary to assess the actual incidence and impact of this condition in boxers.

### Avulsion of the optic nerve

Optic nerve avulsion happens when a relatively small foreign body (eg, a finger) intrudes in the space between the orbital bones and the eye globe.[30–32] Optic nerve head avulsion has been known to occur in contact sports,[33–36] and may be present without obvious evidence of external eye injury.[34] Optic nerve avulsion may be missed in radiologic studies, including computed tomography, magnetic resonance imaging, and ophthalmic ultrasound.[30,37] The majority of patients do not recover useful vision in the affected eye, and many are left unable to perceive light. Due to its very poor visual prognosis, optic nerve avulsion is one of the most dreaded accidental injuries. The hallmark of optic nerve avulsion is sudden loss of vision after a blunt trauma that may be regarded as mild. On fundus examination the site where the optic nerve should be is replaced by a cavity, which may be obscured by retinal and vitreous hemorrhage (**Fig. 8**). Finite element analysis in a computer simulator shows that there are two likely mechanisms responsible for avulsion of the optic nerve. First, a rapid globe rotation causes the greatest stress at the point where the optic nerve inserts into the sclera; and second, a sudden deformation of the globe causes an acute increase in intraocular pressure. The first mechanism seems to the responsible for the traumatic avulsion of the optic nerve, whereas the second is to blame for the damage occurring at the optic nerve head.[37] In real-life situations many more forces that cannot be completely accounted for in a finite-model analysis contribute to this injury. Boxers have been particularly vulnerable to thumbing injuries, but since the introduction of thumbless gloves these injuries have become very rare.

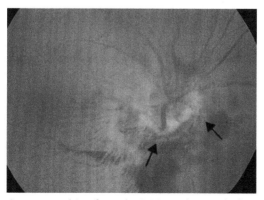

**Fig. 8.** Traumatic optic nerve avulsion from the 3:30- to the 7-o'clock positions (*arrows*).

### Orbital blowout fractures

Blowout fracture has been reported in a 20-year-old amateur boxer who, 15 minutes after a bout, presented complaining of having felt a pop followed by inflation of his left eye after blowing his nose.[38] A study spanning a 20-year period and 1141 blowout fractures in the United States military showed that the most common causes of orbital blowout fractures were violent assault (37.8%), motor vehicle accidents (17.6%), and sports (14.1%).[39] The mechanism of injury involves either (1) transmission of a blow from the thick orbital rim bones to the thin bones of the floor and medial wall of the orbit, which "blow out" and fracture (buckling theory); or/and (2) force transmission from an increase in the intraorbital hydraulic pressure caused by pressure on the eye globe (hydraulic theory). Both mechanisms most likely play a role in this injury. Signs and symptoms include orbital edema, difficulty with eye movements, double vision, enophthalmus, and numbness or tingling of the lower eyelid, nose, and upper lip (V2 branch of the facial nerve, which exits through the inferior orbital fissure in the inferior orbital rim). Sudden orbital swelling or inflating immediately after nose blowing is caused by air being forced from a paranasal sinus (most often the maxillary) to the orbit through a fracture, which may act as a one-way valve, increasing the orbital pressure and potentially leading to a compressive optic neuropathy. Entrapment of the extraocular muscles, particularly the inferior rectus, may lead to ischemia of the muscle and also stimulate a vasovagal reflex, with syncope and bradycardia. Diagnosis is based in history and physical examination, and is confirmed by imaging (computed tomography scan of the orbits with fine cuts). Other injuries should be sought and managed accordingly. Management for blowout fractures may be conservative or surgical.

### SPECIAL CONSIDERATIONS
### Incisional Eye Surgery

Previous incisional eye surgery causes weakness of the eye wall at the site of the incision. The risk of rupture from a blunt injury increases as the size and depth of the incision increase. **Box 1** lists the relative risk of traumatic globe rupture after certain ophthalmic surgeries. Athletes with previous incisional eye surgery should not be allowed to participate in boxing.

### Refractive Surgery in Boxers

Even though at current Food and Drug Administration-approved treatment parameters the eye may not be at higher risk of a rupture than an unoperated eye,[41–43] other complications may occur with blunt trauma. LASIK is a commonly performed refractive procedure in the United States. During the procedure a partial-thickness lamellar flap is created with a microkeratome. Then the flap is lifted and a precalculated pattern of excimer laser is applied to the stromal bed to correct the desired refractive error. The flap is then repositioned to its original position. Studies show that the cornea does not recover its natural, preoperative strength, even after healing is considered to be complete. A study in rabbit corneas found that the cohesive strength of a cornea after a split by blunt dissection was negligible at 5 days, increased rapidly, and leveled at about 100 days with a maximal strength of 25% to 50% of the original.[44] A traumatic dislocation of a LASIK flap may happen at any point after the LASIK procedure, and has been reported as late as 4 years after LASIK surgery (**Fig. 9**).[45] Traumatic loss of the flap may also occur, and has been reported after a karate injury with a finger to the eye 3.5 years after a LASIK procedure.[46] Complications of flap dislocations include epithelial ingrowth infectious keratitis,[47] persistent folds,[48] and irregular

---

**Box 1**
**Predisposition of traumatic ruptured globe after eye surgery**

High

    Penetrating keratoplasty

    Large incision, butt joint cataract extraction

    Radial keratectomy

    Hexagonal keratotomy

Moderately high

    Large incision tapered joint intracapsular cataract extraction, extracapsular cataract extraction (ECCE)

    Trabeculectomy or other filtration surgery

    Prior repair of corneal or scleral laceration

Moderate

    Small incision butt joint ECCE

    "Mini" refractive keratectomy (RK)

    Astigmatic keratectomy

Moderately low

    Small tapered incision ECCE

    Scleral buckle with diathermy

No more than unoperated

    Paracentesis

    Scleral buckle with diathermy

    Strabismus surgery

    Lamellar keratoplasty/pterygium

    Laser in situ keratomileusis (LASIK)

    Photorefractive keratectomy (PRK)

    Keratomileusis

*Data from* Vinger PF. The mechanisms and prevention of sports eye injuries. Available at: http://www.lexeye.com/pdf/Section1.pdf. Accessed August 19, 2009.[40]

---

astigmatism.[48,49] Diffuse lamellar keratitis (inflammation within the corneal interface) may develop as result of mild or significant trauma.[50]

    Due to the high risk of flap trauma in contact sports, boxers should be discouraged from undergoing elective LASIK surgery. Athletes who have already undergone LASIK surgery should be made aware of the potential complications if they decide to practice boxing. Alternative refractive procedures, such as PRK, which do not create a corneal flap, are available and should be preferred over the LASIK procedure.

### Corneal Incisional Surgery (Radial Keratotomy and Hexagonal Keratotomy)

Radial keratotomy and hexagonal keratotomy incisions consists of 90% depth incisions in the corneal stroma. These procedures historically were used to treat astigmatism and myopia, but currently photoablation procedures, like LASIK and PRK, are the preferred method to address these refractive errors. Incisional corneal surgery weakens the corneal structural support. An eye with RK incisions requires about

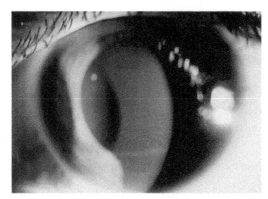

**Fig. 9.** Traumatic flap dislocation with striae. (*From* Nilforoushan M-R, Speaker MG, Latkany R. Traumatic flap dislocation 4 years after laser in situ keratomileusis. J Cataract Refract Surg 2005;31(8):1664–5.   URL:   http://linkinghub.elsevier.com/retrieve/pii/S088633500500177X; with permission.)

half the force to rupture compared with an unoperated eye.[42,51] In the early postoperative period the tensile strength of the cornea may be reduced by 90%, and requires only 25% of the force an intact cornea would require to rupture.[51,52] An unoperated eye usually ruptures at the limbus, behind the rectus muscles insertions, or the lamina cribosa,[53] whereas an eye with RK incisions ruptures at the site of the corneal incisions. Cases of eye rupture through radial keratotomy incisions range from minor (pillow fight) to severe trauma (motor vehicle accident), and their final visual outcome may not correlate with the magnitude of the trauma.[54] Athletes with incisional corneal surgery should not be allowed to participate in boxing, due to the increased risk of rupture at the healed incision site. Modern refractive laser surgery strives to achieve good refractive outcomes without causing structural weakness of the cornea, and should be preferred over incisional surgery.

### Contact Lenses

No contact lenses should be allowed in the boxing ring. Contact lenses can move and dislocate during a fight causing corneal abrasions, foreign body sensation, tearing, and blurring of the vision.

### RISK FACTORS AND PREVENTION

Giovinazzo and colleagues found in a series of 74 boxers that a linear correlation existed between the number of fight losses and the incidence of retinal tears, with 20% prevalence after only 5 losses and 80% prevalence after 40 losses. These investigators also found a steady increase in the probability of retinal tears associated with increased number of bouts, with a 90% probability after 75 bouts.[3] Controversy remains as to whether a boxer with a previously successfully treated retinal detachment should be allowed to continue fighting. Some physicians advocate that eyes with previous laser retinopexy may have stronger retinal attachments than the nonlasered retinas, and are at less risk of suffering a retinal detachment if a retinal tear were to occur.[55] This statement has not been validated in any clinical studies.

To prevent thumbing injuries, thumbless gloves should always be worn while boxing. The New York State Athletic Commission made thumbless boxing gloves mandatory in 1982 for all 4-, 6-, and 8-round bouts.[56]

Functionally one-eyed athletes should not be permitted to participate in boxing activities. For practical purposes, a functionally one-eyed athlete may be defined as having a best-corrected visual acuity worse than 20/40 in the poorer-seeing eye.[57] In this situation, if vision were to be compromised in the better-seeing eye, the athlete may be severely handicapped and unable to obtain a driving license in many states.[58]

## RECOMMENDATIONS

The American Academy of Ophthalmology has issued a policy statement for reforms in boxing[59] with the following recommendations:

1. Examination of boxers before licensure and then after 1 year, six bouts, or two los- ses, or at the stopping of a fight because of an eye injury, or at the discretion of the ringside physician
2. Mandatory, temporary suspension from sparring or boxing for specific ocular pathology—30 days for a retinal tear and 60 days for a treated retinal detachment, or individualized after consultation with the athletic commission medical advisory board
3. Minimal visual requirements of 20/40 or better in each eye and a full central field of not less than 30° on each eye
4. An ophthalmologist required on each state medical boxing advisory board
5. Thumbless boxing gloves to minimize ocular injuries
6. A National Registry of Boxers for all amateur and professional boxers in the United States that records bouts, knockouts, and significant ocular injuries
7. A program from training and recertifying ringside physicians
8. A uniform safety code

## REFERENCES

1. American Academy of Pediatrics, Committee on Sports Medicine and Fitness, American Academy of Ophthalmology, Public Information Task Force. Protective eyewear for young athletes. Ophthalmology 2004;111(3):600–3.
2. Wedrich A, Velikay M, Binder S, et al. Ocular findings in asymptomatic amateur boxers. Retina 1993;13(2):114–9.
3. Giovinazzo VJ, Yannuzzi LA, Sorenson JA, et al. The ocular complications of boxing. Ophthalmology 1987;94(6):587–96.
4. Enzenauer RW, Montrey JS, Enzenauer RJ, et al. Boxing-related injuries in the US army, 1980 through 1985. JAMA 1989;261(10):1463–6.
5. Fundamentals and principles of ophthalmology, vol. 2. American Academy of Ophthalmology; 2005.
6. Vinger PF, Capao Filipe JA. The mechanism and prevention of soccer eye injuries. Br J Ophthalmol 2004;88(2):167–8.
7. Kroll P, Stoll W, Kirchhoff E. [Contusion-suction trauma after globe injuries]. Klin Monatsbl Augenheilkd 1983;182(6):555–9 [in German].
8. Ross WH. Traumatic retinal dialyses. Arch Ophthalmol 1981;99(8):1371–4.
9. Maguire JI, Benson WE. Retinal injury and detachment in boxers. JAMA 1986; 255(18):2451–3.
10. Wolter JR. Coup-contrecoup mechanism of ocular injuries. Am J Ophthalmol 1963;56:785–96.
11. Hagler WS, North AW. Retinal dialyses and retinal detachment. Arch Ophthalmol 1968;79(4):376–88.

12. Delori F, Pomerantzeff O, Cox MS. Deformation of the globe under high-speed impact: in relation to contusion injuries. Invest Ophthalmol 1969;8(3):290–301.

13. Weidenthal DT, Schepens CL. Peripheral fundus changes associated with ocular contusion. Am J Ophthalmol 1966;62(3):465–77.

14. Vinger PF, Duma SM, Crandall J. Baseball hardness as a risk factor for eye injuries. Arch Ophthalmol 1999;117(3):354–8.

15. Vinger PF. Injury to the postsurgical eye. In: Kuhn F, Pieramici DJ, editors. Ocular Trauma, Principles and Practice. New York: Thieme; 2002. p. 280–92.

16. Pierce J, Reinbold John D Jr, Pastore CM. Direct measurement of punch force during six professional boxing matches. Journal of Quantitative Analysis in Sports 2. Available at: http://www.bepress.com/jqas/vol2/iss2/3/. Accessed August 19, 2009.

17. Reidy JJ, Paulus MP, Gona S. Recurrent erosions of the cornea: epidemiology and treatment. Cornea 2000;19(6):767–71.

18. Sankar PS, Chen TC, Grosskreutz CL, et al. Traumatic hyphema. Int Ophthalmol Clin 2002;42(3):57–68.

19. Walton W, Von Hagen S, Grigorian R, et al. Management of traumatic hyphema. Surv Ophthalmol 2002;47(4):297–334.

20. Blanton FM. Anterior chamber angle recession and secondary glaucoma. a study of the aftereffects of traumatic hyphemas. Arch Ophthalmol 1964;72:39–43.

21. Wolff SM, Zimmerman LE. Chronic secondary glaucoma associated with retrodisplacement of iris root and deepening of the anterior chamber angle secondary to contusion. Am J Ophthalmol 1962;54:547–63.

22. American Academy of Ophthalmology. Glaucoma, vol. 10, American Academy of Ophthalmology, 2005.

23. Bianco M, Vaiano AS, Colella F, et al. Ocular complications of boxing. Br J Sports Med 2005;39(2):70–4.

24. Smith DJ. Ocular injuries in boxing. Int Ophthalmol Clin 1988;28(3):242–5.

25. Sugar AP. Ray Leonard undergoes surgery. Available at: http://news.google.com/newspapers?nid=932&dat=19820510&id=xIELAAAAIBAJ&sjid=uVMDAAAAIBAJ&pg=3868,1035538. Accessed August 19, 2009.

26. Kosmorsky G, Lancione RRJ. When fighting makes you see black holes instead of stars. J Neuroophthalmol 1998;18(4):255–7.

27. American Academy of Ophthalmology. Neuro-ophthalmology, vol. 5, American Academy of Ophthalmology, 2005.

28. Steinsapir KD, Goldberg RA. Traumatic optic neuropathy. Surv Ophthalmol 1994; 38(6):487–518.

29. Lessell S. Indirect optic nerve trauma. Arch Ophthalmol 1989;107(3):382–6.

30. Foster BS, March GA, Lucarelli MJ, et al. Optic nerve avulsion. Arch Ophthalmol 1997;115(5):623–30.

31. Hykin PG, Gardner ID, Wheatcroft SM. Optic nerve avulsion due to forced rotation of the globe by a snooker cue. Br J Ophthalmol 1990;74(8):499–501.

32. Fard AK, Merbs SL, Pieramici DJ. Optic nerve avulsion from a diving injury. Am J Ophthalmol 1997;124(4):562–4.

33. Anand S, Harvey R, Sandramouli S. Accidental self-inflicted optic nerve head avulsion. Eye 2003;17(5):646–7.

34. Chow AY, Goldberg MF, Frenkel M. Evulsion of the optic nerve in association with basketball injuries. Ann Ophthalmol 1984;16(1):35–7.

35. Ciolino JB, Murphy MA. Complete optic nerve avulsion associated with a basketball injury. Med Health R I 2003;86(10):324–5.

36. Sanborn GE, Gonder JR, Goldberg RE, et al. Evulsion of the optic nerve: a clinicopathological study. Can J Ophthalmol 1984;19(1):10–6.

37. Cirovic S, Bhola RM, Hose DR, et al. Computer modelling study of the mechanism of optic nerve injury in blunt trauma. Br J Ophthalmol 2006;90(6):778–83.
38. Karsteter PA, Yunker C. Recognition and management of an orbital blowout fracture in an amateur boxer. J Orthop Sports Phys Ther;36(8):611–8.
39. Shere JL, Boole JR, Holtel MR. An analysis of 3599 midfacial and 1141 orbital blowout fractures among 4426 united states army soldiers, 1980–2000. Otolaryngol Head Neck Surg 2004;130:164–70.
40. Vinger PF. The mechanisms and prevention of sports eye injuries. Available at: http://www.lexeye.com/pdf/Section1.pdf. Accessed August 19, 2009.
41. Peacock LW, Slade SG, Martiz J, et al. Ocular integrity after refractive procedures. Ophthalmology 1997;104(7):1079–83.
42. Campos M, Lee M, McDonnell PJ. Ocular integrity after refractive surgery: effects of photorefractive keratectomy, phototherapeutic keratectomy, and radial keratotomy. Ophthalmic Surg 1992;23(9):598–602.
43. Burnstein Y, Klapper D, Hersh PS. Experimental globe rupture after excimer laser photorefractive keratectomy. Arch Ophthalmol 1995;113(8):1056–9.
44. Maurice DM, Monroe F. Cohesive strength of corneal lamellae. Exp Eye Res 1990; 50(1):59–63.
45. Ramirez M, Quiroz-Mercado H, Hernandez-Quintela E, et al. Traumatic flap dislocation 4 years after LASIK due to air bag injury. J Refract Surg 2007;23(7): 729–30.
46. Tetz M, Werner L, Muller M, et al. Late traumatic LASIK flap loss during contact sport. J Cataract Refract Surg 2007;33(7):1332–5.
47. Kim EK, Lee DH, Lee K, et al. Nocardia keratitis after traumatic detachment of a laser in situ keratomileusis flap. J Refract Surg 2000;16(4):467–9.
48. Norden RA, Perry HD, Donnenfeld ED, et al. Air bag induced corneal flap folds after laser in situ keratomileusis. Am J Ophthalmol 2000;130(2):234–5.
49. Lemley HL, Chodosh J, Wolf TC, et al. Partial dislocation of laser in situ keratomileusis flap by air bag injury. J Refract Surg 2000;16(3):373–4.
50. Dudenhoefer EJ, Vinger PF, Azar DT. Trauma after refractive surgery. Int Ophthalmol Clin 2002;42(3):33–45.
51. Larson BC, Kremer FB, Eller AW, et al. Quantitated trauma following radial keratotomy in rabbits. Ophthalmology 1983;90(6):660–7.
52. Uchio E, Ohno S, Kudoh K, et al. Simulation of air-bag impact on post-radial keratotomy eye using finite element analysis. J Cataract Refract Surg 2001;27(11): 1847–53.
53. Kuhn F, Pieramici DJ. Ocular trauma: principles and practice. Illustrated edition. New York: Thieme; 2002.
54. Vinger PF, Mieler WF, Oestreicher JH, et al. Ruptured globes following radial and hexagonal keratotomy surgery. Arch Ophthalmol 1996;114(2):129–34.
55. McLeod D. Ocular injuries from boxing. BMJ 1992;304(6821):197.
56. Rogers T, Scouting; a safer glove. Available at: http://www.nytimes.com/1983/05/03/sports/scouting-a-safer-glove.html. Accessed May 17, 2009.
57. US Consumer Product Safety Commission. Washington, 2000 Sports and recreational eye injuries.
58. Federal Highway Administration. Manual on uniform traffic control devices or streets and highways. Washington: US Department of Transportation; 1988.
59. American Academy of Ophthalmology, Policy statement: reforms for the prevention of eye injuries in boxing, in: San Francisco: Eye Safety and Sports Ophthalmology Committee, June 23, 1990.

# Disabling Hand Injuries in Boxing: Boxer's Knuckle and Traumatic Carpal Boss

Charles P. Melone, Jr., MD, Daniel B. Polatsch, MD*, Steven Beldner, MD

**KEYWORDS**

- Boxer's knuckle • Sagittal band • Extensor hood
- Carpometacarpal boss • Carpometacarpal joint • Arthrodesis

Owing to constant usage with continual exposure to violent forces, the boxer's hands are exceedingly prone to injury. Numerous reports[1,2] confirm that hand injuries are highly prevalent among both amateur and professional fighters and may in fact constitute a sport-specific epidemic. Foremost among these injuries is disruption of the metacarpophalangeal (MP) joints of the fingers, traditionally termed boxer's knuckle.[3,4] The clenched-fist posture, coupled with the enormous forces generated by punching, render the MP joints or knuckles highly vulnerable to damage. The most frequent and severe type of boxer's knuckle encountered is extensor hood disruption, with derangement of the longitudinal central tendon and the transversely oriented sagittal fibers.[4] In such cases, prompt surgical repair is necessary to restore integrity of this critical extensor unit, prevent irreparable tissue damage, and maintain optimal joint function.

The second most common but less recognized type of hand injury apt to cause major disability among fighters is disruption with destabilization of the carpometacarpal (CMC) joints of the fingers, the so-called carpal boss. The excessive trauma of boxing, repeatedly transmitted from the MP joints to the base of the metacarpals, is apt to destabilize the normally rigid CMC joints. Acute sprains and contusions of these joints usually respond successfully to conservative measures; however, untreated or recurrent injuries are prone to result in progressive CMC instability characterized by painful periarticular bony hypertrophy, joint subluxation, and articular degeneration.[5] For the debilitating traumatic carpal boss, selective CMC joint arthrodesis constitutes optimal treatment.

Department of Orthopaedic Surgery, Albert Einstein College of Medicine, Hand Surgery Center, Beth Israel Medical Center, 321 East 34th Street, New York, NY 10016, USA
* Corresponding author.
*E-mail address:* dpolatsch@chpnet.corg (D.B. Polatsch).

Clin Sports Med 28 (2009) 609–621
doi:10.1016/j.csm.2009.06.004
0278-5919/09/$ – see front matter © 2009 Published by Elsevier Inc.

This article, focusing on recognition and management of the debilitating boxer's knuckle and traumatic carpal boss, reviews the key anatomic features of the MP and CMC joints of the hand and, based on the authors' experience with 47 fighters requiring 54 surgical procedures, describes the pathologic anatomy of these potentially career-ending boxing injuries. Moreover, based on this surgical experience, the article reports operative techniques that have proved successful in most cases. In an effort to enhance safety, emphasis also is placed on prevention of injury. Because sport in general is a major source of injury, preventive measures have become a critical aspect of optimal sports medicine that must be increasingly employed in boxing.

## ANATOMY AND PATHOANATOMY
### The Metacarpophalangeal Joint Extensor Hood Mechanism: Normal Anatomy

The extensor hood of the finger MP joint comprises the stout, longitudinal central tendon and the left substantive, but equally important, transverse peripheral fibers, termed the sagittal bands (**Fig. 1**). Integrity of this mechanism permits unimpaired joint function and due to its considerable shock-absorbing capacity, affords protection to the underlying articular surface. An intact extensor hood is essential to successful boxing, whereas traumatic disruption is apt to cause major dysfunction, and requires prompt detection and restoration of the damaged joint.

The dorsally located extensor digitorum communis crosses the center of the MP joint, stabilized within a soft tissue groove. During flexion and extension of the MP joint this central tendon, having no dorsal or volar attachments, glides freely in a longitudinal direction in line with its terminal insertion at the distal phalanx. The central tendon is stabilized ulnarly and radially by the sagittal bands, which originate from the palmar transverse metacarpal ligament and volar plate. Confirming personal observations,[4,5] Tubiana and Valentin[6] demonstrated that the sagittal fibers attach to the lateral borders of the extensor tendon, with some of the fibers traversing the dorsal aspect of the central tendon and uniting with fibers from the opposite side of the tendon, thereby creating a stabilizing groove for the central tendon. Similarly, Ishizuki,[7] in his anatomic study of the extensor mechanism of the long finger, reported that the sagittal bands are divided into thin superficial and thick deep layers. The superficial layer traverses the dorsal aspect of the extensor tendon and the deep layer lies on both sides of the long extensor, forming a central groove that maintains tendon stability. Deep to and separate from the central tendon and the sagittal bands lies the joint capsule of the MP joint, affording additional protection to the articular surface.

Stability of the extensor mechanism also is augmented by the junctura tendinum, connecting the extensors proximal to the MP joints.[8] Although variations in the number and location of these intertendinous structures are frequent, three distinct junctura usually can be identified. One juncture is apt to connect the index and long finger extensor tendons and is usually fascial in structure. A second juncture usually is present between the long and ring finger extensor tendons and may be ligamentous or fascial. An additional juncture connecting the ring and small finger extensors typically is tendinous. The presence of the juncturae enhances resistance to central tendon subluxation at the MP joint and these juncturae have been reported to be injured in some cases of extensor hood disruption.[9]

The bony configuration of the MP joint is also a contributing factor to central tendon stability. The articular surface of the MP joint consists of the eccentrically rounded head of the metacarpal and the matching concavity of the proximal phalanx. This unique contour of the MP joint articular surface induces an ulnar-deviation posture of the fingers as demonstrated by Hakstian and Tubiana.[10] The most commonly

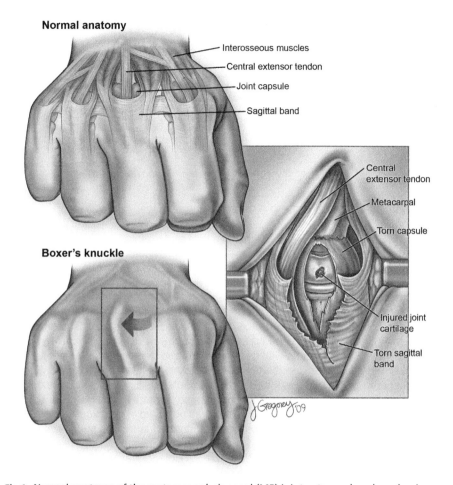

**Fig. 1.** Normal anatomy of the metacarpophalangeal (MP) joint extensor hood mechanism as well as the pathoanatomy of boxer's knuckle. Despite variations in extent and exact location, the characteristic lesion consistently comprised rupture of the sagittal band with subluxation or overt dislocation of the central extensor tendon.

injured index and long finger articular surfaces have a 10° to 15° ulnar inclination whereas the less frequently injured ring and small finger MP joints demonstrate lesser degrees of asymmetry. These investigators infer that this skeletal configuration is an additional element predisposing to instability and displacement of the central extensor tendon when MP joint disruption occurs.

### The Extensor Hood Mechanism: Pathoanatomy

Personal experience with surgical repair of 44 boxer's knuckles, in 38 fighters, reveals consistent patterns of pathology (see **Fig. 1**). Despite variations in extent and exact location, the characteristic lesion consistently comprised rupture of the sagittal band with subluxation or overt dislocation of the central extensor tendon (**Fig. 2**). Twenty-six sagittal bands were ruptured radially, 10 ulnarly, 4 centrally, and 4 completely (radially, centrally, and ulnarly). Similarly, variation occurred with central tendon subluxation, which was usually displaced in the direction opposite the sagittal

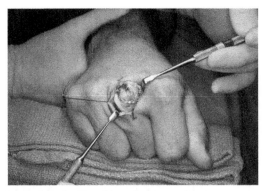

**Fig. 2.** Disrupted extensor hood with subluxed extensor tendon.

band injury. Significantly, 8 of the 10 ulnar sagittal band ruptures were associated with radial subluxation of the central tendon—a lesion previously reported as rare.[11,12] Moreover, in the 4 cases of small finger injury, a major central rupture of the sagittal fibers resulted in an unusual derangement of radial displacement of the extensor digitorum communis tendon and ulnar displacement of the extensor digiti quinti tendon.

Capsular tears were observed in 32 of the 44 MP joints. The tear was invariably located beneath the sagittal band rupture and extended for a variable distance across the joint. In no instance did the capsular injury compromise integrity of the collateral ligaments. However, 5 of the joints with capsular tears also demonstrated osteochondral fractures of the metacarpal head articular surface. Albeit small, ranging from 3 to 10 mm in diameter, these cartilage lesions were characteristically located on the dorsal-central contact area of the metacarpal head, also directly in line with the sagittal band rupture. Notably, all osteochondral fractures occurred in chronic, recurrent, and severely disrupted boxers knuckles, previously untreated or treated nonoperatively.

Without treatment and with repeated trauma to the extensor hood, this relatively thin but critical protective cover of the MP joint clearly deteriorates, exposing the underlying and unsheathed articular surface to an increased risk of chondromalacia, osteochondral fracture, and ultimately degenerative joint disease (**Fig. 3**).

### The Carpometacarpal Joint: Normal Anatomy

The CMC joints of the fingers consist of a complex row of articulations formed by numerous uneven facets on the distal aspect of the distal carpal row connecting

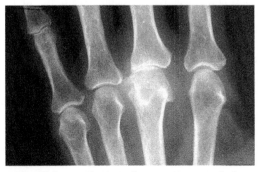

**Fig. 3.** Recurrent, untreated injury to the long finger metacarpophalangeal joint resulting in disabling traumatic arthritis.

with the articular surfaces of the base of the metacarpals.[13] The index metacarpal base articulates mainly through its V-shaped facet with the trapezoid as well as its smaller facets at its radial and ulnar sides that articulate with the trapezium and capitate. The long finger metacarpal articulates via a large triangular facet with the capitate. This configuration creates a snug mortise-and-tenon connection resulting in utmost stability of the index and long finger metacarpals on the distal carpal row, thereby forming the fixed skeletal unit of the hand.

The ring finger metacarpal articulates by a small flat facet with the capitate and by a large quadrilateral facet with the hamate. This configuration permits motion, albeit relatively minor, in the sagittal plane in contrast to the rigid index and long finger CMC joints. The small finger metacarpal articulates through a saddle-shaped facet with the hamate, permitting considerable motion of approximately 20° to 30°.

Numerous palmar and dorsal ligaments contribute to the stability of the CMC joints but have considerable variability in their location and number. The dorsal ligaments are substantially stronger than their palmar counterparts and whereas the index and long finger CMC joints typically have two supporting ligaments, the less stable ring and small finger CMC joints usually have one. Additional stability of the CMC joints is provided by the radial and longitudinal interosseous ligaments spanning the index, long, and ring finger articulations. The intermetacarpal joints located at the base of the 4 metacarpals are stabilized by numerous intermetacarpal and interosseous ligaments that also provide support to the CMC joints, most prominently those of the index and long fingers.

Dynamics stabilizers of the CMC joints include the extensor carpi radialis longus and extensor carpi radialis brevis tendons inserting at the dorsal aspect of the base of the index and long finger metacarpals, respectively; the extensor carpi ulnaris tendon attaching to ulnar aspect of the small finger metacarpal; the flexor carpi ulnaris tendon via its pisometacarpal ligament extension inserting onto the palmar aspect of the small finger metacarpal; and the flexor carpi radialis tendon with its strong attachments to the base of the index and long finger metacarpals.

### The Carpometacarpal Joint: Pathoanatomy

The rigid bony architecture coupled with the substantive static and dynamic soft tissue restraints of the index and long finger CMC joints serve to direct, absorb, and stabilize load transmission from the fingers to the wrist. Nonetheless, with excessive, often violent forces such as those encountered in boxing, CMC instability is apt to occur and result in a major compromise in hand function (**Fig. 4**). With repetitive transmission of pathologic forces from the metacarpals to the CMC joints, periarticular hypertrophic bone spurs develop with concomitant articular subluxation and degeneration. With increasing chronicity, a painful bony mass progressively enlarges at the base of the index and long finger CMC joints, resulting in the classic and disabling traumatic carpal boss (**Fig. 5**).

#### AUTHORS' PREFERRED MANAGEMENT

Most hand injuries in boxing undoubtedly can be successfully managed by nonoperative measures. However, a clear consensus exists that the MP joint extensor hood disruption or boxer's knuckle, and the symptomatic traumatic CMC boss are optimally treated by surgical methods. For these usually chronic and always severe injuries, conservative treatment is an unrealistic option for the competitive boxer whose expectations are a successful recovery with a rapid return to competition.

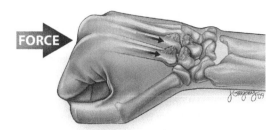

**Fig. 4.** Repetitive transmission of detrimental forces of the MP joints to the carpometacarpal (CMC) joints is prone to cause traumatic carpal boss formation.

### Boxer's Knuckle: Diagnosis and Operative Treatment

These surgical lesions are readily detected by an accurate description of injury, a precise physical examination, and supplemental high-quality radiography. Rarely are specialized imaging studies necessary. Characteristic features of the complete MP joint extensor hood disruption include marked swelling; decreased joint motion, often with an extensor lag; central tendon subluxation, accentuated by flexion of the joint; and a palpable, markedly tender gap at the site of sagittal band rupture. Radiography, including tangential views (Brewerton) of the joint,[14] occasionally demonstrate metacarpal head subchondral cysts, highly suggestive of the occurrence of MP joint osteochondral fracture (**Fig. 6**).

### Operative techniques

In our experience with 38 professional fighters, having incurred 44 boxer's knuckles, regardless of the interval between injury and surgery, direct repair of these lesions has been possible and consistently successful (**Fig. 7**). Because a midline incision directly over the apex of the metacarpal head is apt to result in a painful obtrusive scar with additional impairment, a curved incision, avoiding the prominence of the knuckle, affords preferential exposure. Following extensor tenolysis and sagittal band debridement, the location and extent of soft tissue disruption is clearly visualized. The extensor mechanism is precisely coapted with the joint positioned in 60° to 70° of flexion, permitting a tension-free repair that subsequently will not restrict joint mobility. However, capsular tears, if present, are debrided but not repaired thus

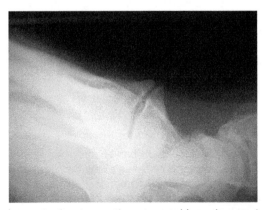

**Fig. 5.** Radiograph demonstrating traumatic metacarpal boss characterized by periarticular hypertrophic spur formation with concomitant articular degeneration.

avoiding an excessively tight soft tissue closure prone to result in a highly detrimental loss of joint flexion. Although some reports[15,16] advocate dorsal capsule repair, the risk of MP joint dysfunction is excessive, whereas without repair no functional deficits have been observed.[4,5] In contrast to capsular tears, osteochondral fractures require precision repair. Debridement and drilling of these lesions, occasionally augmented with capsular flap resurfacing, are critical to promote fibrocartilage ingrowth with preservation of articular integrity. The sagittal bands are repaired with strong, absorbable sutures following which the central tendon is relocated and secured in its midline groove, thereby restoring tendon stability at the extremes of both extension and flexion. Postoperatively the reconstructed joints are immobilized in 60° to 70° of flexion for 6 weeks, following which an intensive program of hand therapy is pursued. Punching is permissible when the knuckle demonstrates thorough wound healing with a pain-free, full arc of motion, and the hand regains near-normal strength, a period of recovery ranging from 8 to 12 weeks.

### Traumatic Carpal Boss: Diagnosis and Operative Treatment

Preoperatively, traumatic CMC boss demonstrates the classic features of a painfully large and tender bony prominence with or without cyst formation overlying the index and long finger CMC joints. Although these digits are the most common sites for traumatic bossing, any or all of the CMC joints may be involved. Tangential radiographs characteristically display hypertrophic bone formation adjacent to, and occasionally overlying, a widened CMC joint space. With increasing chronicity, an enlarging bony mass may completely obliterate degenerative CMC joints.

Our experience includes 9 professional boxers with 11 symptomatic bosses, all of which were treated by CMC joint arthrodesis (**Fig. 8**). In 8 cases the index and long finger CMC joints were the site of fusion, whereas in 3 the arthrodesis included all 4 finger CMC joints. Although wedge resection of the unstable CMC joints has been advocated for painful carpal bossing,[17,18] an inordinate risk of recurrent instability with further joint deterioration[19,20] precludes this procedure as a viable option for the competitive boxer.

### Operative techniques

The CMC joints are approached through a transverse incision directly over the carpal boss (**Fig. 9**). Attention is immediately directed toward identifying and protecting the

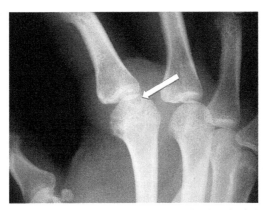

**Fig. 6.** Radiograph demonstrating a subchondral cyst at the head of the index metacarpal highly suggestive of boxer's knuckle associated with osteochondral fracture (*arrow*).

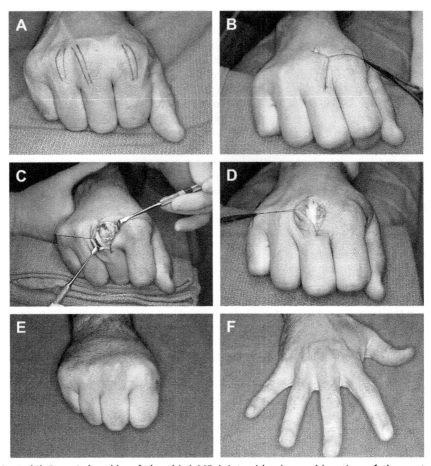

**Fig. 7.** (*A*) Boxer's knuckle of the third MP joint with ulnar subluxation of the central extensor tendon. (*B*) Curved incision over the MP joint. The prominence of the metacarpal head is avoided. (*C*) Surgical pathology. Radial sagittal band disruption with ulnar subluxation of central extensor tendon and underlying capsular tear. The metacarpal head is exposed. (*D*) Radial sagittal band is repaired and the central extensor tendon centralized over the metacarpal head. (*E, F*) Centralized extensor tendon and full active range of motion is achieved postoperatively.

branches of the radial sensory nerve as well as those dorsal cutaneous branches of the ulna nerve.[21] The long digital extensor tendons and the radial wrist extensor tendons are retracted, clearly exposing the carpal boss. The prominent metacarpal bases are visualized and frequently demonstrate subluxation from the adjacent carpal trapezoid, capitate, and hamate articulations. Associated ganglion cysts are excised and subperiosteal dissection exposes the deranged joints. All hypertrophic bone is excised and the involved joints are thoroughly decorticated, completely removing the damaged articular cartilage and subchondral bone. A healthy cancellous trough is created, extending from the radial aspect of the index CMC joint to the ulnar aspect of the most ulnarly affected joint. The thoroughly decorticated and cancellous surfaces of the metacarpals and carpals are precisely coapted and maintained under compression, as multiple 0.062 Kirschner wires are passed percutaneously from the radial

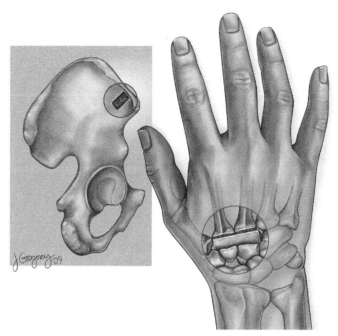

**Fig. 8.** Selective carpometacarpal arthrodesis is performed by placing a cortical cancellous slot graft as well as cancellous autograft, usually procured from the iliac crest, into a precisely created cancellous trough at the involved CMC joints.

aspect of the wrist across the volar aspect of the fusion site, thus affording preliminary stabilization.

A cortical cancellous slot graft along with an abundance of cancellous autograft is then harvested from the outer wall of the iliac crest. The cancellous graft is first inserted and compressed into the trough, ensuring an abundance of healthy bone bridging the fusion site. The slot graft is then carefully sculpted to fit the trough and is first wedged beneath the proximal edge of the metacarpals and then, as the fusion site is distracted, beneath the distal edge of the carpus. The site is then firmly compressed and the insertion of additional 0.062 Kirschner wires ensures secure stabilization. A solid arthrodesis with precise bone graft insertion and accurate wire fixation is confirmed radiographically; the Kirschner wires are bent, cut, and left protruding through the skin.

The capsular tissues are then imbricated and repaired with absorbable sutures. In cases with soft tissue deficiency, a tendon transfer employing the distal half of the insertion of the extensor carpi radialis longus can be advanced dorsally and ulnarly to the insertion of the extensor carpi radialis brevis. The transferred tendon reinforces the capsular tissues and provides not only static but also dynamic stability to the fusion site. The skin wound is closed over a small drain.

The wrist and MP joints are mobilized postoperatively for 6 to 8 weeks or until radiographic union is clearly evident. Once the fusion is solid, the Kirschner wires are removed in the office and an intensive program of hand therapy is initiated. Rehabilitation with alleviation of pain and restoration of mobility and strength sufficient to resume competition requires a period of approximately 6 months.

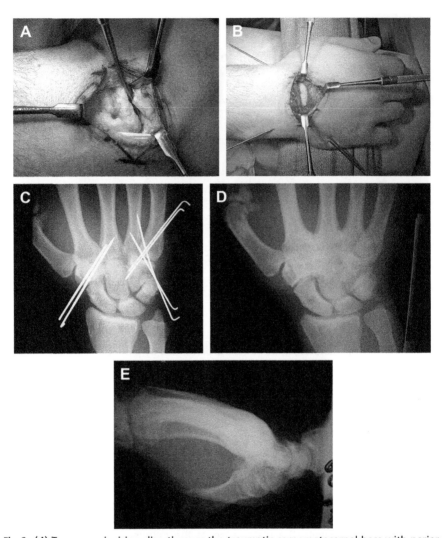

**Fig. 9.** (*A*) Transverse incision directly over the traumatic carpometacarpal boss with periarticular hypertrophic spur formation and concomitant articular degeneration. (*B*) Cortical cancellous slot graft as well as cancellous autograft is compressed into the cancellous trough created at the involved CMC joints. The site is then firmly compressed and the insertion of additional 0.062 Kirschner wires ensures secure stabilization. (*C*) Immediate postoperative radiograph following arthrodesis of all 4 finger carpometacarpal joints. (*D, E*) Postoperative radiographs demonstrating a solid fusion of all 4 finger carpometacarpal joints.

## AUTHORS' ASSESSMENT OF OPERATIVE TREATMENT

For both boxer's knuckle and traumatic carpal boss the outcome of operative treatment has proved consistently favorable. Follow-up evaluation, although difficult to obtain for the competitive boxer, in general has revealed a high level of patient satisfaction, as each athlete experienced relief of pain and recovered digital mobility as well as hand strength commensurate with the needs of a highly competitive boxer, and all returned to unrestricted competition. Three patients initially treated surgically for boxer's knuckle required additional operative procedures. Two required surgery for osteochondral fractures occurring 2 and 4 years, respectively, after their initial operation. Both of these patients experienced a successful treatment regimen and were able to resume their boxing careers. The third boxer, despite uncomplicated surgery for his MP joint, developed a disabling traumatic carpal boss in the ipsilateral hand that was successfully treated by arthrodesis. Subsequently, he also resumed a successful boxing career.

## PREVENTION OF INJURY

Nowhere in sports are the hands at a greater risk for injury than in the boxing ring. Because boxing requires continual exposure of the hands to trauma, boxer's knuckle and traumatic carpal boss are seemingly inevitable consequences. Nonetheless, with recognition of the mechanics as well as the vulnerable sites of injury, preventive measures as applied to other sports can be employed in boxing with an expectant decrease in the occurrence of injury.

Skillful and carefully supervised training is essential to safety. Not only physical conditioning but also hand function should be uncompromised. Flawless, efficient, and potentially less injurious mechanics of punching must be mastered by the fighter, whereas excessive punching should be avoided. Rational methods of taping and wrapping should be precisely contoured to the anatomic configurations of the hand with the objectives of absorbing, diffusing, and diminishing detrimental forces while protecting the vulnerable sites of injury. State boxing commission rules for taping, wrapping, and gloving should be well conceived and carefully formulated with protection as a foremost consideration. Furthermore, commission rules should be standardized so that the hands are continually protected and each fighter is afforded access to beneficial methods of injury prevention.

Custom-fit gloves and flexible casts with increased shock-absorbing capacity are not permissible in boxing matches, but can be provided for training and sparring.[5] Also, the principles of these devices should be incorporated in the design and manufacture of bout gloves as a rational additive measure against detrimental forces incurred by the hand. These protective devices are especially beneficial to the boxer returning to the ring after injury.

The fighter returning from injury requires particularly careful management. Because full recovery is contingent not only on healing of damaged tissues but also on comprehensive rehabilitation of repaired structures, a carefully planned therapy program is essential to a successful outcome. The fighter is continually advised that the recovery of mobility, strength, and endurance essential to a successful competitor is optimally achieved with dedicated rehabilitation that may require several or more months. The fighter also must be continually cautioned against a premature return to competition that is prone to a considerable risk of reinjury.

The boxer's hands should be constantly monitored by knowledgeable medical personnel for pain and other evidence of potentially disabling trauma. Inflammation, bruising, swelling, and tenderness at vulnerable sites are signs of injury that should be thoroughly evaluated and treated before the fighter is permitted to resume punching. When serious injury is either suspected or detected, consultation with sports medicine specialists is advised.

With increasing recognition and application of preventive measures in boxing, the incidence of hand injuries and the need for operative intervention will undoubtedly diminish.

## SUMMARY

The authors advocate operative treatment of the two most debilitating hand-related boxing injuries; namely, boxer's knuckle and traumatic carpal boss. Recognition of the normal anatomy as well as the predictable pathology facilitates an accurate diagnosis and precision surgery. For boxer's knuckle, direct repair of the disrupted extensor hood, without the need for tendon augmentation, has been consistently employed; for traumatic carpal boss, arthrodesis of the destabilized CMC joints has been the preferred method of treatment. Precisely executed operative treatment of both injuries has resulted in an expectant favorable outcome, as in the vast majority of cases the boxers have experienced relief of pain, restoration of function, and an unrestricted return to competition. An increasing application of preventive measures to the sport of boxing should decrease the occurrence of injury and the need for operative intervention.

## ACKNOWLEDGMENTS

We thank Jill K. Gregory, MFA, CMI, Medical Illustrator, for the artwork in **Figs. 1, 4,** and **8.**

## REFERENCES

1. Estwanik JJ, Boitano M, Ari N. Amateur boxing at the 1981 and 1982 USAf ABF national championship. Phys Sportsmed 1984;12:123–8.
2. Jordan BD, Campbell EA. Acute injuries among professional boxers in New York state: a 2-year survey. Phys Sportsmed 1988;16:87–91.
3. Gladden RJ. Boxer's knuckle. A preliminary report. Am J Surg 1957;93:388–97.
4. Hame SL, Melone CP. Boxer's knuckle. Traumatic disruption of the extensor hood. Hand Clin 2000;16(3):375–80.
5. Melone CP. Hand injuries in boxing. In: Jordan BD, editor. Medical aspects of boxing. New York: CRC Press; 1993. p. 277–309.
6. Tubiana R, Valentin P. Anatomy of the extensor apparatus and the physiology of the finger extension. Surg Clin North Am 1964;44:897–918.
7. Ishizuki M. Traumatic and spontaneous dislocation of extensor tendon of the long finger. J Hand Surg Am 1970;15:967–72.
8. Wehbe MA. Junctura anatomy. J Hand Surg Am 1992;17:1124–9.
9. Saldana MJ, McGuire RA. Chronic painful subluxation of the metacarpophalangeal joint extensor tendons. J Hand Surg Am 1986;11:420–3.
10. Hakstian RW, Tubiana R. Ulnar deviation of the fingers. The role of joint structure and function. J Bone Joint Surg Am 1967;49:299–316.
11. Araki S, Ohtani T, Tanaka T. Acute dislocation of the extensor digitorum communis tendon at the metacarpophalangeal joint. J Bone Joint Surg Am 1987;69:616–9.
12. Koniuch MP, Primer CA, VanGorder T, et al. Closed crush injury of the metacarpophalangeal joint. J Hand Surg Am 1987;12:750–7.
13. Yu HL, Chase RA, Strauch B. Atlas of hand anatomy and clinical implications. St. Louis (MO): Mosby; 2004.
14. Lane CS. Detecting occult fractures of the metacarpal head: Brewerton view. J Hand Surg Am 1977;2:131–3.
15. Posner MA, Ambrose L. Boxer's knuckle—dorsal capsular rupture of the metacarpophalangeal joint of a finger. J Hand Surg Am 1989;14:229–35.
16. Pyne JI, Adams BD. Hand tendon injuries in athletics. Clin Sports Med 1992;11: 833–50.

17. Clarke AM, Wheen DJ, Visvanathan S, et al. The symptomatic carpal boss. Is simple excision enough. J Hand Surg Br 1999;24:591–5.
18. Van der Aa JP, Noorda RJ, Van Royen BJ. Symptomatic carpal boss. Orthopedics 1999;22:703–4.
19. Citteur JM, Ritt MJ, Bos KE. Carpal boss: destabilization of the third carpometa-carpal joint after wedge excision. J Hand Surg Br 1998;23:76–8.
20. Vermeulen GM, de With MC, Bleys RL, et al. Carpal boss: effect of wedge exci-sion depth on third carpometacarpal joint stability. J Hand Surg Am 2009;34(1): 7–13.
21. Polatsch DB, Melone CP, Beldner S, et al. Ulnar nerve anatomy. Hand Clin 2007; 23(3):283–9.

# Rehabilitation of Orthopaedic and Neurologic Boxing Injuries

Todd Lefkowitz, DO, Steven Flanagan, MD, Gerard Varlotta, DO, FACSM*

**KEYWORDS**

• Boxing • Rehabilitation • Injuries • Orthopaedic • Neurological

Clinical decision making for injured boxers follows the same therapeutic principles as the treatment plan for other injured athletes. Just as advances in surgical techniques have improved, so has the scientific basis for implementing therapeutic exercises progressed to create an optimum continuum of care and return the athlete to their former level of competition.

## ORTHOPAEDIC REHABILITATION

Most orthopaedic injuries in boxing can be approached in the same manner as other sporting injuries. The principles of PRICE (protection, rest, ice, compression, and elevation) guide treatment for most common musculoskeletal injuries, such as strains and sprains. The initial phase of rehabilitation treatment is to control inflammation. Medications, injections, therapeutic modalities, and rest can all be used to help the inflammation subside so injured boxers can perform an adequate rehabilitation program. Acute fractures and dislocations, although rare in professional and amateur boxing, can often be treated with splinting or casting, or may require surgical intervention.

Athletes progress through three phases of rehabilitation. The first phase is designed to restore pain-free active range of motion (AROM). The second phase works on stabilization and strengthening exercises. The final phase incorporates sport-specific training exercises to help athletes return to their preinjury state of competition. This article focuses on the rehabilitation of orthopaedic injuries common to boxing, with most attention given to shoulder and knee injuries because which these represent the two most debilitating injuries in boxing.

Department of Rehabilitation Medicine, New York University School of Medicine, Rusk Institute of Rehabilitation Medicine, 317 East 34th Street, 5th Floor, NY 100016, USA
* Corresponding author.
*E-mail address:* rustyvarlotta@aol.com (G. Varlotta).

Clin Sports Med 28 (2009) 623–639
doi:10.1016/j.csm.2009.07.002
0278-5919/09/$ – see front matter © 2009 Published by Elsevier Inc.

sportsmed.theclinics.com

## Spinal Rehabilitation

Injuries to the cervical spine are exceedingly rare in professional and amateur boxing. One case of a cervical spine fracture was reported in 1983,[1] followed by a case report of a transient spinal cord injury in a young boxer who had dynamic cervical spine instability and an os odontoideum in 1996.[2] These types of injuries argue for pre- and post-participation screening of the cervical spine, but currently each state's sanctioning body is responsible for conducting its own assessment of professional boxers before and after matches.

Low back pain and injuries to the lumbar spine have not been well documented in boxing medical literature. Jordan and colleagues reported that back injuries accounted for 6.9% of all boxing injuries (447 total) reported over 10-years at the U.S. Olympic Training Center.[10] Preexisting low back pain in the boxer may be exacerbated during running and other roadwork activities used to increase cardiovascular conditioning. A brief period of rest with local heat or ice application, and a short course of nonsteroidal anti-inflammatory drugs (NSAIDs) can be tried. Prolonged NSAID therapy should be avoided, especially if the boxer is training in a warm climate, because the prostaglandin inhibition induced by these medications can promote vasoconstriction and contribute to renal toxicity.

As the acute pain subsides, boxers may incorporate more core stability exercises into the training program. Richardson and Jull described an exercise program to train the cocontraction of the deep trunk muscles (ie, transversus abdominus and lumbar multifidi) to enhance spinal stability in patients who have low back pain.[3] Full abdominal sit-ups and other exercises that may increase intra-abdominal pressure, such as the bench press and military press, may aggravate the low back pain, especially in the presence of an annular tear or herniation, as a concomitant rise in intradiscal pressure occurs. McKenzie-type exercises may be helpful in boxers who experiences radicular symptoms, and should be performed in a directional preference until centralization of the referred spinal pain occurs.[4,5]

Epidural steroids may be necessary if an exercise-based program fails to alleviate symptoms. Nonbony injuries to the cervical spine, such as sprains/strains, herniated intervertebral discs, or whiplash-associated disorders, although not frequently reported, should be suspected in boxers who sustain repeated blows to the head and neck. Rehabilitation of these injuries begins with pain reduction using ice, NSAIDS, and transcutaneous electrical nerve stimulation (TENS) units. Once pain-free AROM is restored, the boxer is instructed on how to perform cervical stabilization exercises, including chin tucks and isometric contractions against resistance.

Cervical traction and manipulation is contraindicated in cases with acutely herniated discs, but may be useful in sprains/strains and whiplash-associated disorders when no signs of neurologic compromise are present.

## Upper Extremity Rehabilitation

Rehabilitation of shoulder injuries in boxing requires quickly restoring pain-free AROM, glenohumeral joint stability, and muscle strength, because the shoulder is the base of support for throwing powerful punches. Experienced boxers often sustain overuse impingement-type injuries,[6] whereas novice boxers, especially military boxers, are prone to musculotendinous strains, subluxations, and dislocations.[7,8]

In the absence of a glenohumeral dislocation that requires closed reduction and a brief period of sling immobilization, most boxers who sustain impingement-type injuries of the rotator cuff can begin immediate postinjury rehabilitation once pain and inflammation have decreased. Stick-and-pulley range of motion exercises are instituted in all planes of shoulder motion. The posterior shoulder capsule should be stretched by gently accentuating cross-arm shoulder adduction with the contralateral arm. Stretching a tight pectoralis major muscle may help attain further range of motion from the shoulder external rotators and abductors.

Rotator cuff strengthening exercises should begin as soon as the boxer achieves full shoulder AROM. Rubber bands, pulleys, or light free weights may be used to isolate and help strengthen the four rotator cuff muscles. Supraspinatus strengthening is important to help prevent impingement against the acromion, because the supraspinatus actively depresses the humeral head during abduction of the shoulder. Resisted internal rotation of the shoulder with the arm abducted to 90° preferentially strengthens the infraspinatus muscle, whereas rotating the shoulder out against resistance with the elbow flexed to 90° and locked to the boxer's side helps strengthen the teres minor.

Periscapular muscle strengthening exercises must be incorporated into the boxer's rehabilitation program because they help stabilize the glenohumeral joint. Shoulder shrugs strengthen the superior fibers of the trapezius muscle, and may be performed with the addition of a weight bar. The serratus anterior and rhomboid muscles can be strengthened with various push-up exercises. Boxers should progress from wall push-ups to knee push-ups to regular push-ups, as muscle strength and endurance increases. The latissimus dorsi is strengthened with shoulder press-up exercises or lat pull-downs performed with a weight bar and pulley.

The treatment of first-time traumatic glenohumeral dislocations in boxers has not been systematically studied. These injuries result from explosive missed punches in boxers who lack adequate glenohumeral stability and upper extremity strength. The boxer's shoulder can be immobilized for comfort, but range of motion exercises with external rotation to neutral should begin as soon as tolerated.[9] The training staff must avoid overstretching the static ligamentous stabilizers of the boxer's shoulder that could further destabilize the joint. As with other contact sports, surgical stabilization of the shoulder may be considered initially if the boxer wishes to continue competing.[10]

The repetitive punches thrown in competition and training places great stress across the elbow joints of boxers, resulting in cumulative microtrauma. Ulnar collateral ligament sprains and tears may be seen initially. Posterior elbow impingement may result from continued hyperextension and pronation of the forearm during rapid punching drills. This injury was recently termed *boxer's elbow* and is associated with osteophyte formation on the posterolateral aspect of the olecranon on arthroscopy.[11] It has been described as the opposite of the valgus extension overload syndrome seen in overhead throwing athletes.[11]

Injuries to the elbow may require a period of relative rest to aid tissue healing. Ultrasound and iontophoresis may be useful adjuncts because the injured structures about the elbow are superficial. A neoprene elbow sleeve may be worn for comfort and proprioception. AROM of the elbow is usually quickly restored because intraarticular pathology of the elbow is rare from boxing injuries. Boxers should be counseled to avoid hyperextension triceps exercises because these may continue to irritate the olecranon and exacerbate elbow impingement. Failure of nonoperative management is an indication for arthroscopy to shave down any osteophytes on the olecranon.

Injuries to the wrist and hand are covered extensively in other articles in this issue, but the general principles of hand rehabilitation are worth mentioning. The most common injuries to the hands in boxing are soft-tissue cuts and abrasions, which rarely require treatments more than simple aseptic first aid. Repeated trauma to the metacarpal phalangeal (MCP) joints, proximal interphalangeal (PIP) joints, and distal interphalangeal (DIP) joints can cause painful hyperkeratotic, fissured callosities known as *boxers' knuckle pads*.[12] These occupational marks can be prevented with proper padding in the glove, and topical emollients and moisturizers.

Hypertrophy of the carpometacarpal joints at the base of the index and middle fingers can be a cause of chronic hand pain in many boxers. The pain from metacarpal bossing can be treated initially with various physical therapy modalities. Fluidotherapy, paraffin baths, and whirlpool treatments are advantageous to boxers because they can enhance AROM of the wrist and hand as the tissues are heated. Once pain has decreased, added protection of the hand is usually necessary for boxers to continue sparring or competing.

### Lower Extremity Rehabilitation

Lower extremity injuries in the boxer, especially those affecting the knee, can be particularly debilitating, because boxing is a weight-bearing sport. Knee injuries are reported to be the second most debilitating injury in boxing aside from shoulder injuries.[13,14]

Agility drills that promote speed and accuracy of punching may aggravate patellofemoral problems. Quadriceps muscle imbalance and patella laxity may predispose boxers to patellofemoral subluxation. Short-arc terminal extension exercises to strengthen the vastus medialis obliquus muscle can help stabilize a subluxing patella, along with a neoprene sleeve or patella taping for additional support. Full range of motion exercises, such as squats that place excessive contact forces between the center of the patella and the trochlea, may exacerbate pain if performed too early.

Physical therapy should address weak primary hip flexors and tight hip abductors as contributing factors to continued patellofemoral problems. Other biomechanical issues in the boxer, such as pes planus and hyperpronation at the subtalar joint, can be addressed with custom-molded orthotics to help normalize lower extremity kinetics.

Patella and quadriceps tendonitis may respond to a brief period of rest with cessation of weight-bearing exercises. These injuries are often associated with jogging and jumping rope during training.[6]

Local ultrasound treatment and topical NSAID preparations may be helpful because the inflamed tissues are superficial. Corticosteroid injections are generally discouraged because they may predispose to rupture of the extensor mechanism of the knee. A patella compression strap (ie, Chopart's strap) may be more helpful than a knee sleeve to help rest the injured tendon, in the same manner as a tennis elbow brace helps rest the radial wrist extensors' tendinous insertion in lateral epicondylitis.

Meniscal tears in the boxer can initially be managed conservatively with PRICE. An intraarticular corticosteroid injection may be used to quickly reduce inflammation and pain. A larger effusion that interferes with AROM should be drained by way of an arthrocentesis before corticosteroid instillation.

In the absence of mechanical symptoms, boxers can progress from range of motion exercises to quadriceps- and hamstring-strengthening exercises. Mechanical symptoms, such as catching or locking of the knee, may require arthroscopic debridement or repair. Meniscal repair has a reported failure rate between 10% and 30%.[15] Like other athletes, boxers who return to training or competition too soon after arthroscopy may jeopardize their surgical repair.

A single strain of the medial head of the gastrocnemius muscle was reported in one series of amateur boxers.[13] Rehabilitation of these injuries is similar to quadriceps or hamstring strains/partial tears. PRICE principles apply and may require application of an elastic bandage to limit bleeding into the muscle. After the initial pain and swelling subsides, gentle stretching exercises are begun followed by an ice massage. A calf sleeve can be used for additional support. Boxers should be counseled to avoid running, jumping, and other push-off activities for 4 to 6 weeks or until pain-free.

In the same series of amateur boxers, one lateral ankle sprain was reported.[13] Rehabilitation of a lateral ankle sprain begins with the boxer being placed in an air cast for comfort and support. Depending on the severity of the sprain, the boxer's lace-up ankle boot may suffice to limit swelling and protect from additional injury. Achilles' tendon stretching and strengthening of the dynamic ankle stabilizers (ie, dorsiflexors and evertors) is encouraged.

Reestablishing motor control with ankle proprioception exercises is of paramount importance for preventing reinjury. Working on a balance board helps retrain the ligament feedback mechanism so boxers can feel comfortable again performing various agility drills without looking down at their feet. Functional conditioning is the last component of the ankle rehabilitation program and incorporates running on curves (figure of eights) and zigzag running with cutting.

In summary, the goals of a rehabilitation program are to reverse or prevent the adverse sequelae of disuse or immobilization and to facilitate tissue healing while avoiding excessive stress on immature tissues. These goals can be achieved by controlling inflammation, progressively increasing mobility, progressively strengthening all muscle groups in the kinetic chain, and maintaining conditioning of uninjured areas. A functionally based rehabilitation program enables athletes to return to full and optimal participation in their sport. Knowledge of the details of the sport's demands, implementation of a motor learning component, and sport-specific training must be incorporated into the rehabilitation program for a successful return to the physically demanding sport of boxing.

## NEUROLOGIC REHABILITATION
### Cognitive Problems and Treatment

Cognitive problems often result from traumatic brain injury and can be a significant barrier to successful participation in desired societal roles. Concussion-related cognitive impairments are known to result from participation in sporting events.[16–26] How long these impairments last is unclear, primarily because of methodological and design problems of the studies examining this issue, including lack of adequate controls and insensitive outcome measures.[17,26–28] What is known, however, is that repetitive concussions, as may occur from boxing, result in impaired cognition.[29–33]

Cognitive problems that do not spontaneously resolve within several months require formal assessment and intervention. Treatment has traditionally focused on two broad areas: remediation techniques that help people develop compensatory strategies using relatively preserved cognitive abilities, and pharmacologic interventions that attempt to improve skills through enhancing specific neurotransmitter systems involved in cognitive function.

Cognitive remediation techniques vary depending on the skills addressed. Regardless of the specific impairment being treated, many techniques have been developed and studied that have the goal of improving a person's ability to function using relatively well-preserved cognitive skills that compensate for identified weaknesses. In this sense, the goal is not to reacquire lost cognitive skills, but rather to help people learn techniques that assist them to function despite their impairments. Approaches to ameliorate the impact of impaired attention, memory, and executive skills have been well studied. Although the quality of the studies varies considerably, substantial evidence on the effectiveness of some modalities exists to provide treatment recommendations in the form of practice guidelines or standards.[34,35]

For example, Attention Process Training (APT) has been shown to be a beneficial means to improve self-reports of attention and memory, and improve objective measure of executive skills. It involves tasks that use specific domains in attention, such as divided, sustained, selective, and alternating attention. Increasing demands are placed on attention skills as individuals progress through training.[36] Other approaches using increasingly challenging tasks that require incorporation of working memory also have been shown to improve attention.[37]

For individuals who have slow processing speed and experience information overload in daily tasks, time pressure management is another effective modality used to train them to compensate for their impairment in real-life tasks.[38] Because of these and other studies,[39,40] strategy planning is recommended as a practice standard to address attention deficits after brain injury.[35]

Memory problems are among the most common complaints after TBI, regardless of injury severity. Several remediation strategies using compensatory techniques have been shown to be useful in improving function. In a group of subjects who had mild memory impairments, visual imagery was shown to be more effective in improving delayed recall of everyday relevant information than standard memory therapy that relied on calendars and notebooks.[41] This technique was also noted to be effective by relatives of the subjects being trained, with improvements lasting up to 3 months postintervention.[41]

Diary use has helped ameliorate the effect of impaired memory on daily function. Studies have shown that diary use combined with a self-instructional training program that teaches individuals to use a strategy to improve daily functioning resulted in more consistent use of the diary and fewer reports of memory problems than diary use alone. The self-instructional training component of this technique provided greater ecologic validity to individuals who had memory problems than task-specific training that focused solely on how to use the dairy.[42]

Other remediation techniques use technologies, such as paging systems, that are designed to improve independent living for people who have impairments in memory and executive skills. One well-designed study showed that patients using a pager system performed important everyday tasks with significantly greater success over baseline performance.[43]

These and other studies have shown that specific interventions can be used to lessen the adverse impact that impaired memory has on daily function.[35] However, specific interventions seem better suited for specific memory problems or severity of impairment. For example, visual imagery has shown efficacy in ameliorating the effect of impaired verbal recall,[41] whereas external memory aids seem useful even in persons many years after injury.[42] Although these two approaches seem best suited to individuals who have milder memory impairments, technologic modalities such as pager system can be useful for those who have more severe impairments, even when other techniques have been ineffective.[43]

Executive function, which can be described as an integration of several cognitive processes that people rely on to regulate and manage goal-directed activities, is also commonly affected after brain injury. As with other cognitive impairments, several techniques have been shown to effectively remediate its impact on daily activities. Goal management training is a structured interactive manual-based rehabilitation protocol that trains people to achieve daily goals despite distractions. It has been shown to improve the completion of goal-oriented tasks in subjects who have TBI.[44]

Other techniques, such as training individuals to break down problems into manageable steps, have been shown to improve the ability to plan and organize better than training geared to improve memory.[45] This approach also improved self-awareness of brain injury–related deficits, goal-directed ideas, and problem-solving abilities, and reduced impulsivity, which is another common post-TBI problem,[45] reflecting the generalization of the results. As a result of these studies, formal problem-solving strategy training has been recommended as a means to address executive-skill dysfunction resulting from brain injury.[35]

A comprehensive and holistic approach to treat cognitive dysfunction involves interventions that address several impaired domains within an integrated and systematic paradigm. These interventions typically are provided within the context of a day treatment program, with evidence suggesting they can improve community reintegration, social participation, and productivity for individuals with moderate to severe brain injury.[46–49] These interventions have also shown to be effective for individuals who are more than 1 year postinjury,[47] with sustained benefits noted long after the intervention ceased.[46,50,51] Therefore, they have been recommended as a practice guideline for people with cognitive impairments after moderate to severe brain injury.[34–51]

### Pharmacologic enhancement of cognitive skills

Some clinicians choose to use medications to improve cognitive skills after TBI. Although a growing body of literature supports their effectiveness, little is class I evidence. Therefore, their use for this purpose remains off-label and no standards of care exist for their use. Clinicians who choose to prescribe medications to enhance cognitive performance after brain injury must critically assess and judiciously use available information to logically approach treatment. They must have a basic understanding of the currently known neurophysiologic and neuroanatomic basis of cognition and the results of clinical trials.

### Attention

Normal attention is mediated in frontal and parietal lobe networks that receive input from ascending catecholaminergic and cholinergic pathways.[52] Pharmacologic interventions aimed at improving attention have focused on enhancing the noradrenergic and cholaminergic neurotransmitter systems.

Many studies in TBI have examined methylphenidate, which is a noradrenergic agonist. It has been found to consistently improve processing speed,[53–55] which seems to be independent of its effect on motor speed.[56] Other studies also support its desirable effect on several other aspects of attention,[57,58] although it has not been well established as a means to improve vigilance, sustained attention, or distractibility.[55,59] Existing evidence has prompted the recommendation of methylphenidate as a treatment guideline to improve attention after TBI.[60]

Although not as well studied as methylphenidate for its impact on attention, acetylcholine agonists have also been examined post-TBI. Most studies have focused on acetylcholinesterase inhibitors, which are currently approved to improve memory in people who have dementia. Donepezil,[61–63] glanatamine,[62] and rivastigmine[62] have all been shown in small trials to improve attention after TBI. Donepezil is currently recommended as a treatment guideline to improve attention after TBI.[60]

### Memory

Acetylcholine has long been implicated in normal learning and memory.[64] Unsurprisingly, its depletion has been shown in several disease states that are manifested by impaired memory. Its role in cognition has also been indirectly assessed by examining the adverse effects of anticholinergic agents that have been shown to cause sedation, confusion, delirium, cognitive decline, and psychotic symptoms in individuals who have Alzheimer's disease.[65]

Many studies have examined the potential role of acetylcholinergic agonists to improve post-TBI memory deficits. Unfortunately, most of these studies had considerable methodological problems that limited their conclusions and generalization.[66] One notable exception is a well-designed study examining rivastigmine in individuals who had varying degrees of memory impairment, which failed to show improvement in memory when all subjects were included in the analysis. However, a subgroup analysis showed that individuals who had the most severe impairment realized a benefit.[67]

### Executive function

Various amphetamines, such as methylphenidate, dextroamphetamine, and guanfacine, have been shown to improve executive function in healthy adults,[68–71] This finding has led to studies examining the potential role of catecholaminergic agonists in subjects who have TBI. Bromocriptine, a dopamine agonist with specificity for the $D_2$ receptor, was found to improve mental flexibility and task performance involving initiation in subjects who had severe TBI,[72] and its use has been recommended as a treatment guideline to improve executive skills in patients who have severe TBI.[60] Accordingly, just as catecholaminergic agonists improve cognitive skills, the use of catecholaminergic antagonists must be restricted after TBI whenever possible. Impaired cognitive functioning has been associated with antipsychotic medication, particularly in those that are potent $D_2$ receptor blockers, such as haloperidol.[73,74] Additionally, the adverse effects of catecholamine blockade on other brain injury–related impairments, such as motor and language function, must also be considered. Retrospective evidence suggests that many commonly used drugs, including catecholamine antagonist, can impair motor and functional recovery after ischemic brain injury.[75]

### Behavior problems

Behavioral disturbances caused by TBI are numerous, and include problems such as agitation, aggression, depression, apathy, and anxiety. They often adversely impact the ability of clinicians to provide effective rehabilitation interventions, and frequently become chronic problems. Similar to the impact imposed by cognitive impairments, altered behaviors are a frequent cause of limited social participation for people who have TBI. They are a considerable source of concern for clinicians treating these patients, and to family members who are often poorly prepared to effectively deal with loved ones who manifest challenging behaviors.

The underlying causes of impaired behavior post-TBI are many and must be accounted for when developing intervention strategies. Alterations in neurotransmitter function, cognitive impairments, poorly adaptive environments, and inappropriate demands on patient performance will collectively worsen behaviors and must therefore be addressed if meaningful change is to occur. Depending on the specific problem, multiple treatment options are often used, including environmental and behavioral modifications; education of clinicians, patients, and loved ones; and medications.

### Agitation/Aggression

#### Behavioral strategies

Agitation and aggression are among the most troublesome problems for clinicians and loved ones after TBI. These terms are frequently used interchangeably and often refer to different behaviors, such as restlessness, causing considerable confusion. Therefore, it is best to specify particular behaviors, rather than provide a generic label. Effectively treating an agitated individual who has TBI requires a comprehensive approach that begins with a careful assessment of the individual and their environment. TBI often exacerbates preexisting personality traits and psychiatric conditions. Identifying strategies used in the past may also provide similar results after TBI-induced exacerbations.

Because preventing agitation is preferable to treating it, identifying antecedents to agitation and initiating strategies to minimize their emergence is important. Antecedents may include exacerbation of comorbid medical problems, such as musculoskeletal injuries that cause pain and lead to agitation. The identification and treatment of these conditions will lessen the appearance of undesired behaviors.

Cognitive impairments may also trigger agitation if the environment is poorly adapted to the person's unique needs, or the demands of expected performance exceed their capabilities. For example, performance expectations exceeding what a cognitively impaired person can reasonably achieve leads to frustration and disappointment, possibly culminating in agitation. This fact must be conveyed to everyone involved in the patient's daily life, because well-meaning individuals may inadvertently initiate agitation by encouraging patients to perform functions they clearly cannot do or cannot do well.

The environment in which the patient functions must also be adapted to their specific needs. For example, an environment full of visual, tactile, or auditory distractions may disenable a person's ability to function adequately, leading to frustration and possible agitation.

Effectively changing behaviors requires an interdisciplinary approach that involves the efforts of the entire rehabilitation team and all individuals involved in the patient's daily life. An effective plan includes the identification and quantification of specific behaviors, both before and during the interventions, and a willingness to provide the necessary time to effect a change, assess its usefulness, and modify the approach as needed.

Strategies to limit the emergence of agitation remain a foundation of any behavioral plan. Behavioral modification uses the thoughtful provision of positive reinforcements and the removal of negative reinforcements. This strategy must be applied consistently by everyone involved in the patient's daily life, because consistency in behavior modification is a key to success. Although the temptation may exist to punish maladaptive behaviors by either removing something deemed desirable or providing something viewed as unpleasant, this is generally believed to do little to alter behaviors in the long-term.[76]

### Pharmacologic treatment of behavior problems

Medications are frequently used to ameliorate behavior problems after TBI. However, unlike many psychiatric conditions in which the use of pharmaceuticals is evidenced-based, a marked paucity exists of well-designed studies examining medication efficacy for individuals who have TBI-related aggression. Therefore, no standards of care or widely accepted guidelines exist on their use to address this problem.[77] In fact, a recent review of the literature found no firm evidence supporting the efficacy of pharmacologic agents in decreasing post-TBI agitation.[78] However, this lack of evidence is likely because of the paucity of well-designed studies, and therefore does not necessarily indicate that commonly used drugs are ineffective.

Several other factors must be considered when prescribing medications for agitation, including the impact a medication will have on other TBI-related comorbidities. Impairments in arousal, cognition, and motor control are well-known sequelae of TBI. However, Yet many drugs used to decrease agitated behavior, such as neuroleptics, benzodiazepines, and anticonvulsants, often worsen these problems. Clearly, clinicians must minimize the use of interventions that may worsen comorbid problems and negatively impact overall function. Many experts also believe that individuals who have TBI are more sensitive to medications than are other populations, making dosing more challenging.[79,80] Furthermore, although medications may be effective in reducing aggression, some may achieve this by primarily decreasing arousal, a potentially troubling effect given that lethargy is a very common post-TBI complaint. Many medications also may have a paradoxic effect, and may exacerbate the very behavior that required modification.

Despite the frequent occurrences of both depression and anxiety after TBI, surprisingly little data supports the effectiveness of medications to treat them. Tricyclic antidepressants (TCAs), specifically amitriptyline[81,82] and desipramine,[83] have been shown to have some effectiveness in decreasing TBI-related depression, although they may be less effective in people who have brain injury than in those without,[82] and often have unacceptable side-effects.[83,84] Sertraline, a selective serotonin reuptake inhibitor, was found to be helpful in decreasing depression in people who have mild TBI,[85–87] although the lack of both a control group and blinding limited the strength of this study.[60] The little existing evidence, however, supports the use of TCAs and serotonin reuptake inhibitors as options for treating post-TBI depression,[60] but note that TCAs may have unacceptable side effects. No conclusive recommendations can be made regarding the pharmacologic treatment of TBI-related anxiety because of the paucity of adequate studies examining this problem.[60]

Slightly more evidence supports the use of certain medications to lessen agitation post-TBI, but again not enough data are available to support a standard of care. Beta-blockers have the strongest evidence for either decreasing the intensity[68] or frequency[83,84] of agitated behavior. This finding has been supported by several other case reports,[88–92] together supporting the use of beta-blockers as a treatment guideline for post-TBI agitation.[60] However, treatment with beta-blockers can be limited by bradycardia and hypotension.[93] Other evidence weakly supports the use of methylphenidate,[94] antidepressants,[85,95–97] valproic acid,[98] lithium,[99–101] and buspirone[102,103] as treatment options.[60]

### Movement disorders

Movement disorders, manifested by abnormalities such as tremors, dystonia, myoclonus, dyskinesias, and Parkinsonism, occur frequently after TBI, although more often as a consequence of severe rather than mild or moderate injuries.[104] However, as many as 10% of people who have mild to moderate TBI experience either a transient or persistent movement disorder, the most common being various types of tremors, which may adversely impact their ability to function.[105] The appearance of a movement disorder may be delayed posttrauma, particularly after repetitive trauma. Parkinsonism resulting from boxing is a classic example of delayed onset, with reports indicating that it manifests several years after the completion of a long boxing career. Repetitive direct blows to the head that apply acceleration and rotational forces to the brain cumulatively occur in boxers who have long careers, and have been associated with the development of Parkinsonism. Symptoms of Parkinsonism have been reported in 20% to 50% of professional boxers, which seems to correlate with the length of time involved in the sport and the number of professional bouts in which they have participated.[106] It is often accompanied by other problems, such as dysarthria, hypophonia, behavioral changes, cognitive decline, and tremors.[104]

Effective treatment of chronic unremitting post-TBI movement disorders is challenging, and often not satisfying. Medication management has been suggested to decrease tremors, including the use of benzodiazepines, anticholinergics, beta-blockers, anticonvulsants, and dopaminergic agonists, although their effectiveness was reported in case series and is otherwise poorly studied.

Radiofrequency lesions of the thalamus have been reported,[107] but although they seem effective in reducing tremors, notable surgical risks are associated that often include worsening of dysarthria and gait abnormalities, preventing this procedure from becoming widely used in this population.[104,107] Results of case reports examining deep brain stimulation indicate that this technique may be effective for ameliorating posttraumatic tremors, without the complications associated with thalamotomy.[108–110] However, more studies must be conducted. Therefore, standard rehabilitation techniques to enhance function and adaptive aids remain the most widely used modalities to treat movement disorders.

### Balance and vestibular disorders

Complaints of dizziness, impaired balance, and a sense of unsteadiness are common after TBI, and occur from several TBI-related morbidities. These occurrences are related to the fact that balance function is controlled by multiple systems, both within and outside of the central nervous system. Peripheral causes of balance dysfunction include benign paroxysmal positional vertigo (BPPV), labyrinthine concussion, temporal bone fracture, and perilymphatic fistula. Central causes of impaired balance include injuries to the brain stem and cerebellum, whereas psychological conditions such as anxiety can also exacerbate the sensation of imbalance, contributing to clinical complaints.[111]

BPPV is among the most common causes of post-TBI dizziness and is manifested by brief episodes of vertigo produced by head movements. It is caused by displacement of crystals from the otoliths into the semicircular canals and is typically transient. BPPV can be easily assessed using the Dix-Hallpike maneuver, with a positive test indicated by inducement of either nystagmus or the sensation of vertigo. Successful treatment may only require the use of canalith reposition procedures that move crystals out of the semicircular canal.[112–114]

Labyrinthine concussions are theorized to occur from violent movement of tissues and fluids in the inner ear and from cell death.[111] It is manifested by sudden-onset hearing loss and vertigo after trauma. The symptoms are generally transient and last from several seconds to several minutes. Individuals who have labyrinthine concussions are usually good candidates for vestibular and balance rehabilitation, using various techniques. Although medications to suppress symptoms may be useful in some cases, they are generally avoided because they delay the natural compensatory processes that naturally follow trauma-induced vestibular dysfunction, and may also impede the rehabilitation process.

Temporal bone fractures may also cause both impaired hearing and vestibular dysfunction. Symptoms caused by longitudinal fractures are usually self-limited, although transverse fractures that involve the otic capsule or internal auditory canal cause more severe hearing loss and vertigo. CT imaging specifically for the temporal bone is required to properly assess the nature of the fracture, because standard head CT scans and radiographs provide insufficient imaging data.

Cranial nerves VII and VIII are vulnerable to injury with temporal bone fractures, which can contribute to hearing loss and balance problems. Traumatic perilymphatic fistulas arise most commonly from an external force that causes injury to the oval window. It is manifested clinically by sudden-onset hearing loss, tinnitus, and vertigo posttrauma and may be aggravated by changes in pressure. It is typically a diagnosis of exclusion because no definitive diagnostic test exists other than direct observation through endoscopy. Treatment is conservative and includes limited bed rest, head elevation, and avoidance of straining. Surgical correction is rarely required.

Medications, including antihistamines, anticholinergics, phenothiazine, and benzo-diazepines have also been used to treat post-TBI vestibular problems. However, they often have unacceptable side effects, including lethargy and confusion, and should therefore be avoided whenever possible after TBI. Surgical intervention is rarely required for perilymphatic fistula and temporal bone fractures when symptoms remain unremitting or worsen despite implementation of more conservative measures. The mainstay of treatment is vestibular and balance rehabilitation that uses specific exercises to promote habituation to stimuli that previously caused vertigo. Other rehabilitation techniques include exercises that promote vestibular adaptation and adoption of alternate strategies that promote effective eye movements.

## REFERENCES

1. Strano SD, Marais AD. Cervical spine fracture in a boxer—a rare but important sporting injury. A case report. S Afr Med J 1983;63:328–30.
2. Place HM, Ecklund JM, Enzenauer RJ. Cervical spine injury in a boxer: should mandatory screening be instituted? J Spinal Disord 1996;9(1):64–7.
3. Jordan BD, Voy RO, Stone J. Amateur boxing injuries at the US Olympic Training Center. Phys Sportsmed 1990;8:81–90.
4. Welch MJ. Few head injuries in academy boxing study. Phys Sportsmed 1982; 10:43–4.
5. Welch MJ, Sitler M, Kroeten H. Boxing injuries from an instructional program. Phys Sportsmed 1986;14:81–90.
6. Mellion MB, Putukian M, Madden CC. Sports medicine secrets. 3rd edition. Hanley & Belfus, Inc, Medical Publishers; 2003.
7. Hardy P, Thabit G, Fanton GS, et al. Arthroscopic management of recurrent anterior shoulder dislocation by combining a labrum suture with antero-inferior holmium: YAG laser capsular shrinkage. Orthopade 1996;25:91–3.
8. Valkering KP, van der Hoeven H, Pijnenburg BCM. Posterolateral elbow impingement in professional boxers. Am J Sports Med 2008;36(2):328–32.
9. Kanerva L. Knuckle pads from boxing. Eur J Dermatol 1998;8(5):359–61.
10. Richardson CA, Jull GA. Muscle control—pain control. What exercises would you prescribe? Man Ther 1995;1(1):2–10.
11. May S, Donelson R. Evidence-informed management of chronic low back pain with the McKenzie method. Spine J 2008;8:134–41.
12. Long, Donelson R, Fung T, et al. Does it matter which exercise? A randomized controlled trial of exercise for low back pain. Spine 2004;29:2593–602.
13. Porter M, O'Brien M. Incidence and severity of injuries resulting from amateur boxing in Ireland. Clin J Sport Med 1996;6:97–101.
14. Gambrell RC. Boxing: medical care in and out of the ring. Curr Sports Med Rep 2007;6:317–21.
15. Greene WB. Essentials of musculoskeletal care. 2nd edition. American Academy of Orthopaedic Surgeons; 2001.
16. Collins P, Roberts AC, Dias R, et al. Perseveration and strategy in a novel spatial self-ordered sequencing task for nonhuman primates: effects of excitotoxic lesions and dopamine depletions of the prefrontal cortex. J Cogn Neurosci 1998;10:332–54.
17. Cremona-Meteyard SL, Geffen GM. Persistent visuospatial attention deficits following mild head injury in Australian Rules football players. Neuropsychologia 1994;32:649–62.

18. Echemendia RJ, Putukian M, Mackin RS, et al. Neuropsychological test performance prior to and following sports-related mild traumatic brain injury. Clin J Sport Med 2001;11:23–31.
19. Hinton-Bayre AD, Geffen G. Severity of sports-related concussion and neuropsychological test performance. Neurology 2002;59:1068–70.
20. Hinton-Bayre AD, Geffen G, McFarland K. Mild head injury and speed of information processing: a prospective study of professional rugby league players. J Clin Exp Neuropsychol 1997;19:275–89.
21. Hinton-Bayre AD, Geffen GM, Geffen LB, et al. Concussion in contact sports: reliable change indices of impairment and recovery. J Clin Exp Neuropsychol 1999;21:70–86.
22. Lovell MR, Collins MW. Neuropsychological assessment of the college football player. J Head Trauma Rehabil 1998;13:9–26.
23. Lovell MR, Collins MW, Iverson GL, et al. Recovery from mild concussion in high school athletes. J Neurosurg 2003;98:296–301.
24. Macciocchi SN, Barth JT, Alves W, et al. Neuropsychological functioning and recovery after mild head injury in collegiate athletes. Neurosurgery 1996;39: 510–4.
25. Maddocks D, Saling M. Neuropsychological deficits following concussion. Brain Inj 1996;10:99–103.
26. Matser EJ, Kessels AG, Lezak MD, et al. Neuropsychological impairment in amateur soccer players. JAMA 1999;282:971–3.
27. Bleiberg J, Cernich AN, Cameron K, et al. Duration of cognitive impairment after sports concussion. Neurosurgery 2004;54:1073–8 [discussion: 1078–80].
28. Tysvaer AT, Storli OV, Bachen NI. Soccer injuries to the brain. A neurologic and electroencephalographic study of former players. Acta Neurol Scand 1989;80: 151–6.
29. Ravdin LD, Barr WB, Jordan B, et al. Assessment of cognitive recovery following sports related head trauma in boxers. Clin J Sport Med 2003;13:21–7.
30. Ross RJ, Casson IR, Siegel O, et al. Boxing injuries: neurologic, radiologic, and neuropsychologic evaluation. Clin Sports Med 1987;6:41–51.
31. Casson IR, Siegel O, Sham R, et al. Brain damage in modern boxers. JAMA 1984;251:2663–7.
32. Drew RH, Templer DI, Schuyler BA, et al. Neuropsychological deficits in active licensed professional boxers. J Clin Psychol 1986;42:520–5.
33. Kaste M, Kuurne T, Vilkki J, et al. Is chronic brain damage in boxing a hazard of the past? Lancet 1982;2:1186–8.
34. Cicerone KD, Dahlberg C, Kalmar K, et al. Evidence-based cognitive rehabilitation: recommendations for clinical practice. Arch Phys Med Rehabil 2000;81: 1596–615.
35. Cicerone KD, Dahlberg C, Malec JF, et al. Evidence-based cognitive rehabilitation: updated review of the literature from 1998 through 2002. Arch Phys Med Rehabil 2005;86:1681–92.
36. Sohlberg MM, McLaughlin KA, Pavese A, et al. Evaluation of attention process training and brain injury education in persons with acquired brain injury. J Clin Exp Neuropsychol 2000;22:656–76.
37. Cicerone KD. Remediation of "working attention" in mild traumatic brain injury. Brain Inj 2002;16:185–95.
38. Fasotti L, Kovacs F, Eling PA, et al. Normal 0 Time pressure management as a compensatory strategy training after closed head injury. Neuropsychol Rehabil 2000;10:47–65.

39. Novack TA, Caldwell SG, Duke LW, et al. Focused versus unstructured intervention for attention deficits after traumatic brain injury. J Head Trauma Rehabil 1996;11:52–60.

40. Gray JM, Robertson I, Pentland B, et al. Microcomputer based attentional retraining after brain damage: a randomized group controlled trial. Neuropsychol Rehabil 1992;2:97–115.

41. Kaschel R, Della Sala S, Cantagallo A, et al. Imagery mnemonics for the rehabilitation of memory: a randomised group controlled trial. Neuropsychol Rehabil 2002;12:127–53.

42. Ownsworth TL, Mcfarland K. Memory remediation in long-term acquired brain injury: two approaches in diary training. Brain Inj 1999;13:605–26.

43. Wilson BA, Emslie HC, Quirk K, et al. Reducing everyday memory and planning problems by means of a paging system: a randomised control crossover study. J Neurol Neurosurg Psychiatry 2001;70:477–82.

44. Levine B, Robertson IH, Clare L, et al. Rehabilitation of executive functioning: an experimental-clinical validation of goal management training. J Int Neuropsychol Soc 2000;6:299–312.

45. von Cramon DY, von Cramon M, Mai N. Problem solving deficits in brain injured patients. A therapeutic approach. Neuropsychol Rehabil 1991;1: 45–64.

46. Sander AM, Roebuck TM, Struchen MA, et al. Long-term maintenance of gains obtained in postacute rehabilitation by persons with traumatic brain injury. J Head Trauma Rehabil 2001;16:356–73.

47. Seale GS, Caroselli JS, High WM Jr, et al. Use of community integration questionnaire (CIQ) to characterize changes in functioning for individuals with traumatic brain injury who participated in a post-acute rehabilitation programme. Brain Inj 2002;16:955–67.

48. Malec JF. Impact of comprehensive day treatment on societal participation for persons with acquired brain injury. Arch Phys Med Rehabil 2001;82:885–95.

49. Klonoff PS, Lamb DG, Henderson SW, et al. Outcome assessment after milieu-oriented rehabilitation: new considerations. Arch Phys Med Rehabil 1998;79: 684–90.

50. Klonoff PS, Lamb DG, Henderson SW. Outcomes from milieu-based neurorehabilitation at up to 11 years post-discharge. Brain Inj 2001;15:413–28.

51. Klonoff PS, Lamb DG, Henderson SW. Milieu-based neurorehabilitation in patients with traumatic brain injury: outcome at up to 11 years postdischarge. Arch Phys Med Rehabil 2000;81:1535–7.

52. Coull JT. Neural correlates of attention and arousal: insights from electrophysiology, functional neuroimaging and psychopharmacology. Prog Neurobiol 1998;55:343–61.

53. Gualtieri CT, Evans RW. Stimulant treatment for the neurobehavioural sequelae of traumatic brain injury. Brain Inj 1988;2:273–90.

54. Mahalick DM, Carmel PW, Greenberg JP, et al. Psychopharmacologic treatment of acquired attention disorders in children with brain injury. Pediatr Neurosurg 1998;29:121–6.

55. Whyte J, Hart T, Schuster K, et al. Effects of methylphenidate on attentional function after traumatic brain injury. A randomized, placebo-controlled trial. Am J Phys Med Rehabil 1997;76:440–50.

56. Whyte J, Hart T, Vaccaro M, et al. Effects of methylphenidate on attention deficits after traumatic brain injury: a multidimensional, randomized, controlled trial. Am J Phys Med Rehabil 2004;83:401–20.

57. Kim YH, Ko MH, Na SY, et al. Effects of single-dose methylphenidate on cognitive performance in patients with traumatic brain injury: a double-blind placebo-controlled study. Clin Rehabil 2006;20:24–30.
58. Plenger PM, Dixon CE, Castillo RM, et al. Subacute methylphenidate treatment for moderate to moderately severe traumatic brain injury: a preliminary double-blind placebo-controlled study. Arch Phys Med Rehabil 1996;77:536–40.
59. Speech TJ, Rao SM, Osmon DC, et al. A double-blind controlled study of methylphenidate treatment in closed head injury. Brain Inj 1993;7:333–8.
60. Neurobehavioral Guidelines Working Group, Warden DL, Gordon B, et al. Guidelines for the pharmacologic treatment of neurobehavioral sequelae of traumatic brain injury. J Neurotrauma 2006;23:1468–501.
61. Khateb A, Ammann J, Annoni JM, et al. Cognition-enhancing effects of donepezil in traumatic brain injury. Eur Neurol 2005;54:39–45.
62. Tenovuo O. Central acetylcholinesterase inhibitors in the treatment of chronic traumatic brain injury-clinical experience in 111 patients. Prog Neuropsychopharmacol Biol Psychiatry 2005;29:61–7.
63. Zhang L, Plotkin RC, Wang G, et al. Cholinergic augmentation with donepezil enhances recovery in short-term memory and sustained attention after traumatic brain injury. Arch Phys Med Rehabil 2004;85:1050–5.
64. Hagan JJ, Alpert JE, Morris RG, et al. The effects of central catecholamine depletions on spatial learning in rats. Behav Brain Res 1983;9:83–104.
65. Lu CJ, Tune LE. Chronic exposure to anticholinergic medications adversely affects the course of Alzheimer disease. Am J Geriatr Psychiatry 2003;11:458–61.
66. Poole NA, Agrawal N. Cholinomimetic agents and neurocognitive impairment following head injury: a systematic review. Brain Inj 2008;22:519–34.
67. Silver JM, Koumaras B, Chen M, et al. Effects of rivastigmine on cognitive function in patients with traumatic brain injury. Neurology 2006;67:748–55.
68. Mintzer MZ, Griffiths RR. Triazolam-amphetamine interaction: dissociation of effects on memory versus arousal. J Psychopharmacol 2003;17:17–29.
69. Mattay VS, Callicott JH, Bertolino A, et al. Effects of dextroamphetamine on cognitive performance and cortical activation. Neuroimage 2000;12:268–75.
70. Jakala P, Sirvio J, Riekkinen M, et al. Guanfacine and clonidine, alpha 2-agonists, improve paired associates learning, but not delayed matching to sample, in humans. Neuropsychopharmacology 1999;20:119–30.
71. Elliott R, Sahakian BJ, Matthews K, et al. Effects of methylphenidate on spatial working memory and planning in healthy young adults. Psychopharmacology (Berl) 1997;131:196–206.
72. McDowell S, Whyte J, D'Esposito M. Differential effect of a dopaminergic agonist on prefrontal function in traumatic brain injury patients. Brain 1998;121(Pt 6):1155–64.
73. Mysiw WJ, Bogner JA, Corrigan JD, et al. The impact of acute care medications on rehabilitation outcome after traumatic brain injury. Brain Inj 2006;20:905–11.
74. Stanislav SW. Cognitive effects of antipsychotic agents in persons with traumatic brain injury. Brain Inj 1997;11:335–41.
75. Goldstein LB. Common drugs may influence motor recovery after stroke. The Sygen In Acute Stroke Study Investigators. Neurology 1995;45:865–71.
76. Kazdin AE, editor. Behavior modification in applied settings. 6th edition. Belmont (CA): Wadsworth/Thomson Learning; 2001.
77. Gordan WA, Zafonte R, Cicerone K, et al. Traumatic brain injury rehabilitation: state of the science. Am J Phys Med Rehabil 2006;85:343–82.

78. Fleminger S, Greenwood RJ, Oliver DL. Pharmacological management for agitation and aggression in people with acquired brain injury. Cochrane Database Syst Rev 2006;(4):CD003299.
79. Silver JM, Arciniegas DB. Pharmacotherapy of neuropsychiatric disturbances. In: Zasler ND, Katz DI, Zafonte RD, editors. Brain injury medicine: principles and practice. New York: Demos; 2007. p. 963–93.
80. McAllister TW. Neuropsychiatric aspects of TBI. In: Zasler ND, Katz DI, Zafonte RD, editors. Brain injury medicine: principles and practice. New York: Demos; 2007. p. 835–61.
81. Saran AS. Depression after minor closed head injury: role of dexamethasone suppression test and antidepressants. J Clin Psychiatry 1985;46:335–8.
82. Dinan TG, Mobayed M. Treatment resistance of depression after head injury: a preliminary study of amitriptyline response. Acta Psychiatr Scand 1992;85:292–4.
83. Wroblewski BA, Joseph AB, Cornblatt RR. Antidepressant pharmacotherapy and the treatment of depression in patients with severe traumatic brain injury: a controlled, prospective study. J Clin Psychiatry 1996;57:582–7.
84. Santos AB, Ballenger JC. Tricyclic antidepressant triggers mania in patient with organic affective disorder. J Clin Psychiatry 1992;53:377–8.
85. Fann JR, Uomoto JM, Katon WJ. Sertraline in the treatment of major depression following mild traumatic brain injury. J Neuropsychiatry Clin Neurosci 2000;12: 226–32.
86. Brooke MM, Patterson DR, Questad KA, et al. The treatment of agitation during initial hospitalization after traumatic brain injury. Arch Phys Med Rehabil 1992; 73:917–21.
87. Greendyke RM, Kanter DR. Therapeutic effects of pindolol on behavioral disturbances associated with organic brain disease: a double-blind study. J Clin Psychiatry 1986;47:423–6.
88. Elliott FA. Propranolol for the control of belligerent behavior following acute brain damage. Ann Neurol 1977;1:489–91.
89. Mansheim P. Treatment with propranolol of the behavioral sequelae of brain damage. J Clin Psychiatry 1981;42:132.
90. Mattes JA. Metoprolol for intermittent explosive disorder. Am J Psychiatry 1985; 142:1108–9.
91. Ratey JJ, Morrill R, Oxenkrug G. Use of propranolol for provoked and unprovoked episodes of rage. Am J Psychiatry 1983;140:1356–7.
92. Yudofsky SC, Williams DT, Gorman J. Propranolol in the treatment of rage and violent behavior in patients with chronic brain syndromes. Am J Psychiatry 1981;138:218–20.
93. Greendyke RM, Kanter DR, Schuster DB, et al. Propranolol treatment of assaultive patients with organic brain disease. A double-blind crossover, placebo-controlled study. J Nerv Ment Dis 1986;174:290–4.
94. Mooney GF, Haas LJ. Effect of methylphenidate on brain injury-related anger. Arch Phys Med Rehabil 1993;74:153–60.
95. Kant R, Smith-Seemiller L, Zeiler D. Treatment of aggression and irritability after head injury. Brain Inj 1998;12:661–6.
96. Kim KY, Moles JK, Hawley JM. Selective serotonin reuptake inhibitors for aggressive behavior in patients with dementia after head injury. Pharmacotherapy 2001;21:498–501.
97. Jackson RD, Mysiw WJ. Abnormal cortisol dynamics after traumatic brain injury. Lack of utility in predicting agitation or therapeutic response to tricyclic antidepressants. Am J Phys Med Rehabil 1989;68:18–23.

98. Wroblewski BA, Joseph AB, Kupfer J, et al. Effectiveness of valproic acid on destructive and aggressive behaviours in patients with acquired brain injury. Brain Inj 1997;11:37–47.

99. Glenn MB, Wroblewski B, Parziale J, et al. Lithium carbonate for aggressive behavior or affective instability in ten brain-injured patients. Am J Phys Med Rehabil 1989;68:221–6.

100. Bellus SB, Stewart D, Vergo JG, et al. The use of lithium in the treatment of aggressive behaviours with two brain-injured individuals in a state psychiatric hospital. Brain Inj 1996;10:849–60.

101. Haas JF, Cope DN. Neuropharmacologic management of behavior sequelae in head injury: a case report. Arch Phys Med Rehabil 1985;66:472–4.

102. Gualtieri CT. Buspirone for the behavior problems of patients with organic brain disorders. J Clin Psychopharmacol 1991;11:280–1.

103. Stanislav SW, Fabre T, Crismon ML, et al. Buspirone's efficacy in organic-induced aggression. J Clin Psychopharmacol 1994;14:126–30.

104. Krauss JK, Jankovic J. Movement disorders after TBI. In: Zasler ND, Katz DI, Zafonte RD, editors. Brain injury rehabilitation: principles and practice. 1st edition. New York: Demos; 2007. p. 469–89.

105. Krauss JK, Trankle R, Kopp KH. Posttraumatic movement disorders after moderate or mild head injury. Mov Disord 1997;12:428–31.

106. Lampert PW, Hardman JM. Morphological changes in brains of boxers. JAMA 1984;251:2676–9.

107. Krauss JK, Mohadjer M, Nobbe F, et al. The treatment of posttraumatic tremor by stereotactic surgery. Symptomatic and functional outcome in a series of 35 patients. J Neurosurg 1994;80:810–9.

108. Broggi G, Brock S, Franzini A, et al. A case of posttraumatic tremor treated by chronic stimulation of the thalamus. Mov Disord 1993;8:206–8.

109. Foote KD, Okun MS. Ventralis intermedius plus ventralis oralis anterior and posterior deep brain stimulation for posttraumatic Holmes tremor: two leads may be better than one: technical note. Neurosurgery 2005;56:E445 [discussion: E445].

110. Umemura A, Samadani U, Jaggi JL, et al. Thalamic deep brain stimulation for posttraumatic action tremor. Clin Neurol Neurosurg 2004;106:280–3.

111. Shepard NT, Clendaniel RA, Ruckenstein M. Balance and dizziness. In: Zasler ND, Katz DI, Zafonte RD, editors. Brain injury: principles and practice. 1st edition. New York: Demos; 2007. p. 491–510.

112. Wolf JS, Boyev KP, Manokey BJ, et al. Success of the modified Epley maneuver in treating benign paroxysmal positional vertigo. Laryngoscope 1999;109:900–3.

113. Parnes LS, Price-Jones RG. Particle repositioning maneuver for benign paroxysmal positional vertigo. Ann Otol Rhinol Laryngol 1993;102:325–31.

114. Herdman SJ, Tusa RJ, Zee DS, et al. Single treatment approaches to benign paroxysmal positional vertigo. Arch Otolaryngol Head Neck Surg 1993;119:450–4.

# Index

*Note:* Page numbers of article titles are in **boldface** type.

## A

Abdominal trauma, blunt, 583–584
   deaths due to, 583
Agent of commission, ringside physician as, 513
Agitation/aggression, following boxing injuries, 630–631
Airborne infections, 547–551
Alcohol, prohibited in competition, 540
Anabolic agents, as prohibited, 536
Anabolic androgenic steroids, as prohibited, 537
Androgenic steroids, anabolic, as prohibited, 537
Angle recession, due to blunt trauma, 596
Antisclerotic disease, 522
Aorta, rupture of, 527
Arrhythmias, 524–525
Attention, boxing injuries and, 629
Auscultation, in valvular disease, 524

## B

ß-Blockers, prohibited in competition, 540–541
Bacterial infections, 553
Balance and vestibular disorders, associated with boxing injuries, 633–634
BALCO, drug concoctions and, 534–535
Behavior problems, boxing injuries and, 630, 631–632
Bloodborne infection, 553–556
Bout, neurologic symptoms following, 565, 566
   reporting results of, Professional Boxing Safety Act of 1996 and, 511
   termination of, ringside physician and, 518
Boxer registry, of Professional Boxing Safety Act of 1996, 509
Boxer(s), bleeding, 580
   medical abnormalities on brain imaging disqualifying, 515
   medical preparticipation evaluation of, ringside physician and, **515–519**
   medical record of, review by ringside physician, 515–517
   prefight medical questions for, 516
   prefight physical examination for, 516–517
   refractive surgery in, 602–603
Boxer's knuckle, diagnosis and operative management of, 614–615, 616
Boxing, and contact sports, cardiovascular issues in, **521–532**
   brain injury in, **561–578**
   eye trauma in, **591–607**
   governing bodies in, 542

Clin Sports Med 28 (2009) 641–648
doi:10.1016/S0278-5919(09)00059-3
0278-5919/09/$ – see front matter © 2009 Elsevier Inc. All rights reserved.

Boxing (*continued*)
    hand injuries in: boxer's knuckle and traumatic carpal boss, **609–621**
    infectious disease and, **545–560**
    medical safety in: administrative, ethical, legislative, and legal considerations,
        **505–514**
    metabolic demand of, 521
    nonneurologic emergencies of, **579–590**
    safety standards in, 579
    specific risks of, 525–528
    status of doping and drug use and, implications for sport, **533–543**
Boxing gym, environment of, contamination of, 546–547
Boxing injuries, agitation/aggression following, 630–631
    attention and, 629
    balance and vestibular disorders associated with, 633–634
    behavior problems and, 630, 631–632
    cognitive skills and, pharmacologic enhancement of, 629
    executive function and, 630
    learning and memory and, 629–630
    movement disorders associated with, 632–633
    neurologic, rehabilitation following, 626–627
    of lower extremity, rehabilitation following, 626–627
    of upper extremity, rehabilitation following, 624–626
    orthopaedic, and neurologic, rehabilitation of, **623–639**
        rehabilitation of, 623
    spinal, rehabilitation following, 624
Boxing match. See *Bout.*
Brain injury, acute traumatic, 561–569
      clinical classification of, 567
      clinical presentation of, 563–565
      concussion and, 564
      diagnosis of, 565
      epidemiology of, 561–562
      management of, 567–568
      pathologic classification of, 562
      pathology of, 565–566
      pathophysiology of, 567, 568
      prevention of, 568–569
      signs and symptoms of, 563
    chronic traumatic, 570–575
      clinical presentation of, 572
      diagnosis of, 573
      epidemiology of, 571–572
      management of, 575
      pathology of, 573–574
      pathophysiology of, 574–575
      prevention of, 575
      risk factors for, 571
    in boxing, **561–578**
    traumatic, assessment for, 518
Bronchitis, 549–550
Brugada syndrome, 587–588

## C

Cannabinoids, prohibition of, 540
Cardiac arrest, in direct blow to chest, 582
Cardiac emergencies, 586–588
Cardiomyopathy(ies), dilated, 523
    hypertrophic, 523
        electrocardiogram to screen for, 528
Cardiovascular abnormalities, recommendations for athletes with, 529
Cardiovascular evaluation of athlete, 528
Cardiovascular events, diagnosis and treatment of, 530
Cardiovascular issues, in boxing and contact sports, **521–532**
Cardiovascular risks of exercise, 522–525
Cardiovascular screening, prebout, 516, 517
Carpal boss, traumatic, diagnosis and operative treatment of, 615–617, 619
Carpometacarpal joint, anatomy of, 612–613
Cataracts, in boxers, 597–598, 599
Chemical and physical manipulation, as prohibited, 539
Chest, blunt trauma to, 581–582
    trauma to, 525
Chylous pericardium, chronic, 527–528
Cognitive skills, following boxing injuries, pharmacologic enhancement of, 629
Common cold, 547
Commotio cordis, 525–527
Congenital heart disease, undiagnosed, 524
Contact infections, 551–553
Contact lenses, 604
Contact sports, and boxing, cardiovascular issues in, **521–532**
Contracoup, to eye, 592–593
Corneal abrasion, 593–594
Corneal incisional surgery, 603–604
Coronary artery anomalies, congenital, 523
Coup injury, to eye, 592
Cyclodialysis, 596

## D

Dehydration, 546
Documentation, of ringside physician, maintenance of, 513–514
Doping, and drug use, status of, implications for boxing, **533–543**
    by athletes, history of, 534
    definition of, 535–536
    substances and methods prohibited, at all times, 536–539
        in competition, 539–540
        in particular sports, 540–541
    World Anti-Doping Agency and, 533, 535
Drug testing, in competition versus out-of-competition, 541–542
Drug use, and doping, status of, implications for boxing, **533–543**
    by athletes, history of, 533–535
Drugs, potentially abused in boxing, 541
    therapeutic use of, exemptions for, 541

**E**

Electrocardiogram, to screen for hypertrophic cardiomyopathies, 528
Emergency preparedness, 588–589
Equatorial expansion, of eye, 592–593
Equipment, safety of, Professional Boxing Safety Act of 1996 and, 511
Ethical guidelines, for ringside physician, 507–509
Executive function, boxing injuries and, 630
Exercise, cardiovascular risks of, 522–525
Eye, rupture of, 593, 594, 595
Eye surgery, incisional, 602
Eye trauma, in boxing, **591–607**
    anatomic considerations in, 592
    incidence of, 591, 599
    mechanisms of, 592
    morbidity associated with, 591
    physics of, 592
    threatening vision, 599
    types of, 593–602
  prevention of, 604–605
  risk factors for, 604

**F**

Fighter. See *Boxer(s)*.
Fighter's contract, indemnification clause in, ringside physician and, 513
Fractures, oribital blowout, 602
Fungus, as cause of infection, 551

**G**

Gene doping, 539
Genital injury, due to blunt trauma, 584
Glasgow coma score, 565, 566, 567
Globe, rupture of, after eye surgery, 603
Glucocorticosteroids, 540
Governing bodies, in boxing, 542

**H**

Hand injuries, in boxing: boxer's knuckle and traumatic carpal boss, **609–621**
  management of, 613–618
  prevention of, 619
Hand(s), anatomy of, 610, 611
  pathoanatomy of, 610–613
  unwrapped, examination of, 518
Heart, adaptations to intense exercise, 522
  anatomy of, 522
Hematoma(s), 580
  subdural, 518
Hepatitis B virus, transmission of, 555–556

Hepatitis C virus, transmission of, 556
Herpes simplex virus skin infection, 552–553
Hormone antagonists and modulators, prohibited, 538
Hormones and related substances, prohibited, 537–538
Human immunodeficiency virus, transmission of, 554–555
Hypertrophic cardiomyopathy, 523, 528
Hyphema, 595–596


I

Identification card, and Professional Boxing Safety Act of 1996, 509–510
Immune system, detrimental effects of exercise on, 546
    physiology of, 545–546
Indian reservations, boxing on, standards and licensing of, 511
Infectious disease, airborne, 547–551
    bloodborne, 553–556
    boxing and, **545–560**
    contact, 551–553
    of upper respiratory tract, 547
Iridodialysis, traumatic, 596, 597
Iritis, traumatic, 595


K

Keratotomy, kexagonal, 603–604
    radial, 603–604
Kidney, injury to, due to blunt trauma, 584


L

Learning and memory, boxing injuries and, 629–630
Legislation of boxing, 509–512
    pending, 512
Legislative guidelines, 509–512
Lens, injury to, in boxers, 597
Liability, strict, doping and, 536
Long QT syndrome, 587
    causes of, 525, 526–527
Lower extremity, injuries in boxing, rehabilitation following, 626–627


M

Macrohyphema, 595, 596
Macula, importance to visual function, 600
Malpractice insurance, ringside physician and, 512–513
Marfan syndrome, 524
Medical abnormalites, on brain imaging, disqualifying fighters, 515
Medical insurance, for ringside physician, maintenance of, 513
Medical issues, exclusion of athletes due to, 529–530
Medical license for jurisdiction of fight, of ringside physician, maintenance of, 513
Medical questions, prefight, 516
        for boxer, 516

Medical requirements, minimum, 506
Metacarpophalangeal joint, extensor hood mechanism of, 610–612
Methicillin-resistant *Staphylococcus aureus* infection, 553
Mitral regurgitation, 524
Movement disorders, associated with boxing injuries, 632–633
MRI scanning, in chronic brain injury, 515
Muhammad Ali Boxing Reform Act, 511
Musculoskeletal system, prefight evaluation of, 517
Myocarditis, 523, 550–551


**N**

Narcotics, prohibition of, 540
Neck, anterior, direct blunt trauma to, 581
Neurologic injuries, in boxing, rehabilitation following, 627–629


**O**

Ocular examinations, of fighters, 515
Ocular injuries, in boxing, 518–519
    vision-threatening, 599
Optic nerve, and visual field defects, 600
    avulsion of, 601
Optic neuropathy, traumatic, 600–601
Oral, ocular, ear/nose/throat trauma, 580–581
Orbital blowout fractures, 602
Orthopedic trauma, in boxing ring, 584–585
Oxygen transfer, enhancement of, as prohibited, 538


**P**

Pericarditis, 549–550
Pharyngitis, 548–549
Physical examination, prefight, for boxer, 516–517
Physician, and Professional Boxing Safety Act of 1996, 509
    ringside. See *Ringside physician.*
Pneumonia, community-acquired, 549
Pre-participation examination, 505–506
Preparticipation screening of athletes, 528
Procedures to be established, Professional Boxing Safety Act of 1996 and, 510
Professional Boxing Safety Act of 1996, 509–511
    boxing registry of, 509
    health, safety, and equipment recommendations of, 511
    identification card and, 510
    physician and, 509
    procedures to be established, 510
    reporting results and, 511
    safety standards of, 509–510
    standards and licensing of, 511
    suspension and, 509

2009 Prohibited List World Anti-Doping Code, 536
Psychotic emergencies, acute, 585


**R**

Retina, peripheral, injury to, 599, 600
Rib fractures, as emergency situation, 582
Ringside physician, 505
    and medical preparticipation evaluation of boxers, **515–519**
    as agent of commission, 513
    documentation by, maintenance of, 513–514
    ethical guidelines for, 507–509
    indemnification clause in fighter's contract and, 513
    legal concerns of, 512–514
    malpractice insurance and, 512–513
    medical insurance for, maintenance of, 513
    medical license for jurisdiction of fight, maintenance of, 513
    post-fight examination by, 507
    requirements of, 579
    review of fighters medical record by, 515–517
    ringside preparticipation by, 506–507
    termination of bout and, 518
Ringside preparation, 506–507


**S**

Safety standards, of Professional Boxing Safety Act of 1996, 509–510
Second impact syndrome, 569–570
Serology, before fight, 516
Sinusitis, acute, 548
Skin infection, herpes simplex virus, 552–553
Spinal injuries, in boxing, rehabilitation following, 624
Spleen, blunt trauma to, 583
*Staphylococcus aureus*, methicillin-resistant infection, 553
Stimulants, prohibition of, 539–540
Subconjunctival hemorrhage, 594–595
Sudden cardiac death, 522, 586–587
Supraventricular arrhythmias, reentrant, 525
Suspension, and Professional Boxing Safety Act of 1996, 509


**U**

Upper extremity, injuries in boxing, rehabilitation following, 624–626
Upper respiratory tract infections, 547


**V**

Valvular disease, 524
Ventricular dysplasia, arrhythmogenic right, 525
Virus, as cause of infection, 551–552

**W**

Warts, 552
Water, for necessary hydration, 546
Weight, stipulated, making of, infection and, 546
World Anti-Doping Agency, 533, 535

**Z**

Zonular trauma, 598–599

# United States Postal Service

## Statement of Ownership, Management, and Circulation
### (All Periodicals Publications Except Requestor Publications)

| 1. Publication Title | 2. Publication Number | 3. Filing Date |
|---|---|---|
| Clinics in Sports Medicine | 0 0 0 - 7 0 2 | 9/15/09 |

| 4. Issue Frequency | 5. Number of Issues Published Annually | 6. Annual Subscription Price |
|---|---|---|
| Jan, Apr, Jul, Oct | 4 | $253.00 |

7. Complete Mailing Address of Known Office of Publication (*Not printer*) (*Street, city, county, state, and ZIP+4®*)

Elsevier Inc.
360 Park Avenue South
New York, NY 10010-1710

Contact Person
Stephen Bushing
Telephone (Include area code)
215-239-3688

8. Complete Mailing Address of Headquarters or General Business Office of Publisher (*Not printer*)

Elsevier Inc., 360 Park Avenue South, New York, NY 10010-1710

9. Full Names and Complete Mailing Addresses of Publisher, Editor, and Managing Editor (*Do not leave blank*)

Publisher (*Name and complete mailing address*)

John Schrefer, Elsevier, Inc., 1600 John F. Kennedy Blvd. Suite 1800, Philadelphia, PA 19103-2899

Editor (*Name and complete mailing address*)

Ruth Malwitz, Elsevier, Inc., 1600 John F. Kennedy Blvd. Suite 1800, Philadelphia, PA 19103-2899

Managing Editor (*Name and complete mailing address*)

Catherine Bewick, Elsevier, Inc., 1600 John F. Kennedy Blvd. Suite 1800, Philadelphia, PA 19103-2899

10. Owner (*Do not leave blank. If the publication is owned by a corporation, give the name and address of the corporation immediately followed by the names and addresses of all stockholders owning or holding 1 percent or more of the total amount of stock. If not owned by a corporation, give the names and addresses of the individual owners. If owned by a partnership or other unincorporated firm, give its name and address as well as those of each individual owner. If the publication is published by a nonprofit organization, give its name and address.*)

| Full Name | Complete Mailing Address |
|---|---|
| Wholly owned subsidiary of | 4520 East-West Highway |
| Reed/Elsevier, US holdings | Bethesda, MD 20814 |

11. Known Bondholders, Mortgagees, and Other Security Holders Owning or Holding 1 Percent or More of Total Amount of Bonds, Mortgages, or Other Securities. If none, check box ☐ None

| Full Name | Complete Mailing Address |
|---|---|
| N/A | |

12. Tax Status (*For completion by nonprofit organizations authorized to mail at nonprofit rates*) (*Check one*)
The purpose, function, and nonprofit status of this organization and the exempt status for federal income tax purposes:
☐ Has Not Changed During Preceding 12 Months
☐ Has Changed During Preceding 12 Months (*Publisher must submit explanation of change with this statement*)

PS Form 3526, September 2007 (Page 1 of 3 (Instructions Page 3)) PSN 7530-01-000-9931 **PRIVACY NOTICE**: See our Privacy policy in www.usps.com

| 13. Publication Title | 14. Issue Date for Circulation Data Below |
|---|---|
| Clinics in Sports Medicine | July 2009 |

| 15. Extent and Nature of Circulation | | | Average No. Copies Each Issue During Preceding 12 Months | No. Copies of Single Issue Published Nearest to Filing Date |
|---|---|---|---|---|
| a. Total Number of Copies (*Net press run*) | | | 1794 | 1623 |
| b. Paid Circulation (By Mail and Outside the Mail) | (1) | Mailed Outside-County Paid Subscriptions Stated on PS Form 3541. (*Include paid distribution above nominal rate, advertiser's proof copies, and exchange copies*) | 1007 | 938 |
| | (2) | Mailed In-County Paid Subscriptions Stated on PS Form 3541 (*Include paid distribution above nominal rate, advertiser's proof copies, and exchange copies*) | | |
| | (3) | Paid Distribution Outside the Mails Including Sales Through Dealers and Carriers, Street Vendors, Counter Sales, and Other Paid Distribution Outside USPS® | 216 | 214 |
| | (4) | Paid Distribution by Other Classes Mailed Through the USPS (e.g. First-Class Mail®) | | |
| c. Total Paid Distribution (*Sum of 15b (1), (2), (3), and (4)*) | | ▶ | 1223 | 1152 |
| d. Free or Nominal Rate Distribution (By Mail and Outside the Mail) | (1) | Free or Nominal Rate Outside-County Copies Included on PS Form 3541 | 84 | 87 |
| | (2) | Free or Nominal Rate In-County Copies Included on PS Form 3541 | | |
| | (3) | Free or Nominal Rate Copies Mailed at Other Classes Through the USPS (e.g. First-Class Mail) | | |
| | (4) | Free or Nominal Rate Distribution Outside the Mail (Carriers or other means) | | |
| e. Total Free or Nominal Rate Distribution (*Sum of 15d (1), (2), (3) and (4)*) | | ▶ | 84 | 87 |
| f. Total Distribution (*Sum of 15c and 15e*) | | ▶ | 1307 | 1239 |
| g. Copies not Distributed (*See instructions to publishers #4 (page #3)*) | | ▶ | 487 | 384 |
| h. Total (*Sum of 15f and g*) | | ▶ | 1794 | 1623 |
| i. Percent Paid (15c divided by 15f times 100) | | | 93.57% | 92.98% |

16. Publication of Statement of Ownership

☐ If the publication is a general publication, publication of this statement is required. Will be printed in the **October 2009** issue of this publication. ☐ Publication not required

17. Signature and Title of Editor, Publisher, Business Manager, or Owner

*Stephen R. Bushing*

Stephen R. Bushing – Subscription Services Coordinator

Date September 15, 2009

I certify that all information furnished on this form is true and complete. I understand that anyone who furnishes false or misleading information on this form or who omits material or information requested on the form may be subject to criminal sanctions (including fines and imprisonment) and/or civil sanctions (including civil penalties).

PS Form 3526, September 2007 (Page 2 of 3)

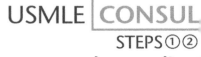

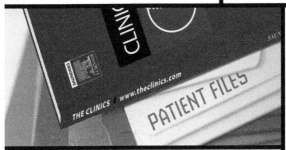

# Moving?

## Make sure your subscription moves with you!

To notify us of your new address, find your **Clinics Account Number** (located on your mailing label above your name), and contact customer service at:

**Email: journalscustomerservice-usa@elsevier.com**

**800-654-2452** (subscribers in the U.S. & Canada)
**314-447-8871** (subscribers outside of the U.S. & Canada)

**Fax number: 314-447-8029**

**Elsevier Health Sciences Division**
**Subscription Customer Service**
**3251 Riverport Lane**
**Maryland Heights, MO 63043**

*To ensure uninterrupted delivery of your subscription, please notify us at least 4 weeks in advance of move.

Printed and bound by CPI Group (UK) Ltd, Croydon, CR0 4YY

03/10/2024

01040464-0008